How the
Brain Grows

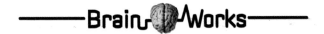

Brain Works

How the Brain Grows

Ann McIntosh Hoffelder, Ph.D.
and
Robert L. Hoffelder, Ph.D.

SERIES EDITOR
Eric H. Chudler, Ph.D.

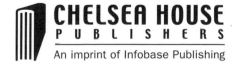

CHELSEA HOUSE
PUBLISHERS
An imprint of Infobase Publishing

To Danielle, Emma, Mack, and Michael, and the young people of their generation,
whose awesome brains are our inspiration and challenge . . .
To those experts in the field of neuroscience and science writing whose research,
experience, and theories laid the foundation . . .

How the Brain Grows

Copyright ©2007 by Infobase Publishing

Chelsea House
An imprint of Infobase Publishing
132 West 31st Street
New York NY 10001

Library of Congress Cataloging-in-Publication Data

Hoffelder, Ann McIntosh.
  How the brain grows / Ann McIntosh Hoffelder and Robert L. Hoffelder.
    p. cm. — (Brain works)
  Includes bibliographical references and index.
  ISBN 0-7910-8946-0 (hardcover)
  1. Brain—Growth—Juvenile literature. I. Hoffelder, Robert L. II. Title. III. Series
  QP376.H66 2006
  612.8'2—dc22   2006017149

Text design by Keith Trego
Cover design by Takeshi Takahashi

Printed in the United States of America

Bang KT 10 9 8 7 6 5 4 3 2 1

This book is printed on acid-free paper.

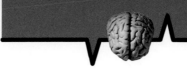

Table of Contents

Introduction

The brain grows—
by leaps and bounds . . .
with ups and downs . . .

The human body is a series of interrelated systems: circulatory and respiratory systems, skeletal and muscular systems, digestive and excretory systems, endocrine and reproductive systems, lymphatic and immune systems, and the nervous system. From its earliest development in the fetus, a complex mass of tissue housed in your skull controls and coordinates these systems, which play out all of your mental and physical actions. This complex mass of tissue is your brain. Your brain is a major part of the nervous system, and without it, none of the other systems could work.

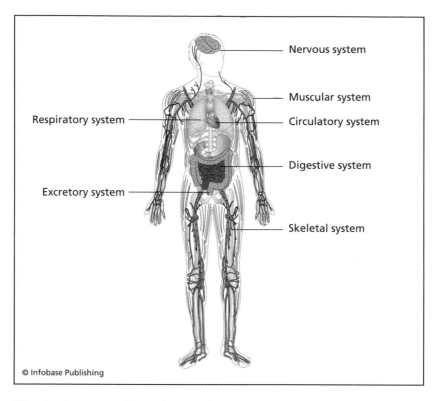

Nervous system

Muscular system

Respiratory system — Circulatory system

Digestive system

Excretory system —

Skeletal system

© Infobase Publishing

The brain controls and coordinates the activity of the various systems of the human body.

Look at your day. Last night, you slept. This morning, you woke up (with or without an alarm or someone pulling you out of bed), ate breakfast (we hope), and went to school. Somehow, along the way, you went through your morning routine, managed to get dressed, and grabbed your books, your homework, and your gym shoes. Lunch, snack, ice cream money . . . you made sure you had everything you needed. You arrived at school and talked to your friends about the usual subjects: "You going to practice after school?" "That was an awesome game last night!" "What have you heard about the school dance this weekend?" And so on, until you heard the bell ring and ran to class.

What was happening in your head that enabled you to do what you usually do almost every day? Where did this brain come from? What is in it? Does it grow? If it grows, how? What affect does its growth have on you? These are questions we will ask and answer in this book. We will also look for how you, and your choices, affect your brain. The following pages will help you visualize, analyze, and appreciate a truly amazing part of yourself—your brain.

CONNECTIONS

The brain does grow, and the "how" is the primary focus of this book. Chapters 1 and 2 will help you establish a visual map of the brain and learn to identify the names and functions of its parts. In Chapter 3, we will look at the connections the brain makes as it communicates within itself and throughout the whole body. In making these connections, the brain grows.

This foundation, in both vocabulary and understanding of the structure, functions, and communication processes of the brain, begins your journey. You will be able to recognize more clearly the different parts of the brain, what they do, and how they do it.

Throughout all of the chapters, we will see how the brain grows—how it begins, develops, and expands in size and complexity. We will see how it changes from when we are babies to our teenage years and beyond. To explain these topics, in Chapter 4 we will follow the prenatal development of the brain and its evolutionary history. Then we will discuss the growth and development of the brain from birth through the teen years (Chapters 5 through 7).

Chapter 8 takes a peek into the future—the hopes and dreams for brain discoveries that might soon be possible. And we will look at some of the research and the achievements that are going on right now that may help us better understand how the brain operates.

1

Structure and Function of Your Brain—Part 1

The strong, bony protective part of the brain is the cranium. It surrounds the brain like a permanent, exclusively designed bike helmet. The cranium's rounded design gives it great strength and the zigzag edges of the bones fit together more firmly than would straight edges. The skin of the scalp covers the cranium bones on the outside, so the places where the bones come together, the **sutures**, are usually not visible.

Three layers of tissue below the cranium provide additional protection for the brain (Figure 1.1). These special layers are called the **meninges**. The outer layer of the meninges is the **dura mater** (or **dura**). It is tough and thick, gives the brain good support, and restricts the brain's movement within the skull. The dura protects

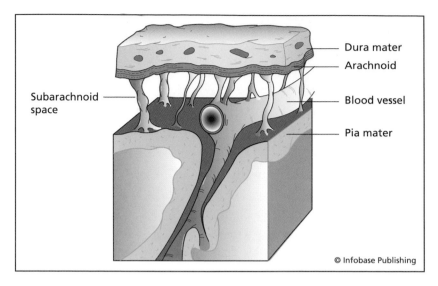

Subarachnoid space

Dura mater
Arachnoid
Blood vessel
Pia mater

© Infobase Publishing

Figure 1.1 The meninges covers the surface of the brain. It consists of three different layers: the dura mater, arachnoid, and pia mater.

the brain from movements that may stretch and break brain blood vessels.

The middle layer of the meninges is the **arachnoid**. (Arachnoid comes from the Greek word meaning "cobweb-like.") Spaces within this layer contain **cerebrospinal fluid (CSF)** and cobweb-like connections to the innermost **pia mater** (or **pia**) layer. The spaces and fluid of the arachnoid layer provide more cushioning for the brain. The CSF circulates around the brain, through the **ventricle** spaces in the brain, and around the spinal cord.

The pia mater is the inner layer of the meninges, the layer closest to the brain. This layer contains the many blood vessels that nourish the brain. The pia is a thin layer and clings to the folds, bumps, and wrinkles of the brain's

Protect the Fortress

Each year, about 2 million Americans suffer brain injuries from some sort of head trauma, impairing their movements, thoughts, and/or bodily functions. Some of the most common causes of brain injury and death are accidents involving cars and motorcycles, sports, and falls. But there are ways to protect yourself. A study of bicycle injuries published in the *Journal of the American Medical Association* reported that wearing bike helmets reduced the risk of head and brain injury by 65% to 70%.

surface—rather like plastic wrap clings to a chunk of raw chopped meat.

A blow to the head or hard shaking, especially of a baby or small child, can really damage the brain. Hard blows, no matter how old you are, can damage your brain; this is why you wear a helmet when you ride your bike or take part in contact sports like football. All of these safeguards are important, because underneath these layers of protection—the bony cranium, and the meninges, the CSF—lies the control center for your whole life: the brain itself.

A GLOBAL VIEW OF THE BRAIN

If you could see the human brain beneath its bony cranial protection, you would see a convoluted, wrinkled, ropy looking, pinkish-gray mass that looks something like a large, mushy walnut. This is the **cerebrum** (Figure 1.2). The outer covering of the cerebrum is the **cerebral cortex**. It is somewhat gray in

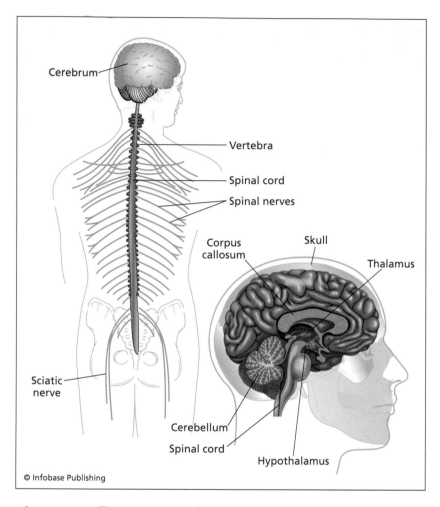

Figure 1.2 The cerebrum is the largest portion of the human brain. It is divided into two hemispheres that are connected by the corpus callosum.

color, which is where the term *gray matter* comes from. The word *cortex* comes from the Latin word for "bark" (as found on a tree) or rind (like the skin around a grapefruit).

The cortex is the outer layer of the brain, and is made up of **neurons** or nerve cells and **glial cells** (neuroglia). Neurons are the impulse- or message-conducting cells of the brain. The **glia** form the supporting structure for the neurons and provide them with nourishment and insulation. The cerebral cortex also has a lot of bulges or ridges (**gyri**) and grooves (**sulci**). The cerebral cortex folds and loops in and out, permitting it to fit into the smaller area of the skull. The total surface area of adult cerebral cortex is about 324 square inches, or the size of a newspaper page flatted out.

The cerebrum is split into two halves by a deep, longitudinal groove. The two halves are designated as the right and left **hemispheres**. These two cerebral hemispheres communicate with each other over a thick bundle of nerve fibers called the **corpus callosum**. The corpus callosum is not wireless like your cell phone. It has a huge mass of nerve fibers, about 200 million of them. This information superhighway can be compared to the Internet, as it networks to connect everything.

The two hemispheres look like mirror images of one another, but they are not. The different hemispheres—in fact, different sections within the hemispheres—handle completely different tasks. However, they must work together, and this teamwork is why the corpus callosum is so important. Imagine it like this: On a basketball or football team, the different players may be assigned specific positions, but they help out in other areas, sometimes even covering for a teammate. To play the game effectively, all the players must work together as a team, so communication—on a sports team as well as in the brain—is tremendously important. We will consider details of how the brain communicates in Chapter 3.

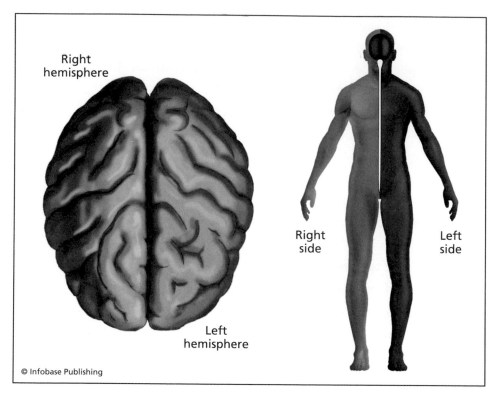

Right
hemisphere

Right
side

Left
side

Left
hemisphere

© Infobase Publishing

Figure 1.3 The right hemisphere of the brain controls muscles on the left side of the body, while the left hemisphere of the brain controls muscles on the right side of the body.

For most people, language, mathematical, and analytical abilities seem to be handled predominately in the left hemisphere. Generally, the right hemisphere handles artistic and musical abilities, abstract reasoning, and manipulating things in space.

It is interesting to note that signals from these hemispheres to the various areas of the body "cross over" in their connections (Figure 1.3). Your right cerebral hemisphere primarily controls the left side of your body, and the left cerebral hemisphere primarily controls the right side of your body. When there is damage to one hemisphere, it affects the opposite side of the body as well as the functions associated with the damaged hemisphere. Sometimes, if one hemisphere is injured, the other hemisphere can reorganize itself to take on some of the tasks of the injured side, depending on the severity of the injury and the age at which the injury occurs.

THE BRAIN'S DIVISION OF LABOR

In order for the brain's activities to run more effectively and efficiently, jobs are divided up. Just as there are different tasks handled by the two hemispheres, there is further specialization within the hemispheres. Each hemisphere is divided into four **lobes**—a frontal lobe, a parietal lobe, an occipital lobe, and a temporal lobe (Figure 1.4). The frontal lobes, located directly behind the forehead, are involved in language, motor skills (including speech and voluntary movements), and cognitive or thought functions. In the frontal lobes, thoughts are transformed into words and words into speech. The control of voluntary movements such as throwing a baseball or playing the piano uses connections originating in the frontal lobes. Actions involving conscious control, such as planning a schedule, presenting a reasoned argument, or solving a problem are functions of the frontal lobes. These actions are called "executive functions."

The parietal lobes lie just behind the **motor area** of the frontal lobes toward the top of the cerebrum. Parietal lobes receive and process sensory input such as touch, pain, temperature, taste, and texture from all parts of the body. One of the ridges of the parietal lobe is concerned with somatic sensation (bodily sensations). This strip of neural tissue is

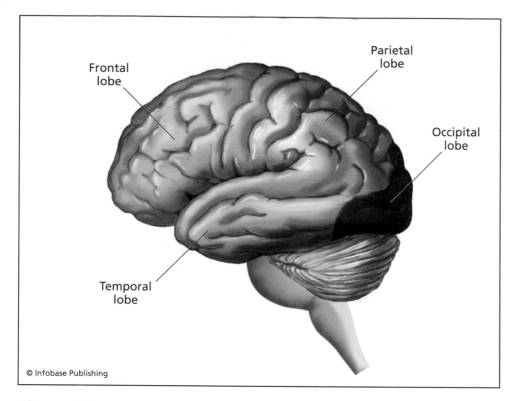

Frontal
lobe

Parietal
lobe

Occipital
lobe

Temporal
lobe

© Infobase Publishing

Figure 1.4 Each hemisphere of the brain consists of four separate sections known as lobes.

referred to as the somatic sensory (somatosensory) cortex and is situated adjacent to the motor cortex of the frontal lobe. For simplicity, we shall refer to this strip of tissue as the sensory cortex.

The occipital lobes are at the back of the brain behind the parietal lobes and above the cerebellum. These lobes are the primary areas for receiving and processing visual information from the eyes. The number of different modules of visual information, such as color, shape, location, and direction of motion, are each processed by distinct regions.

The temporal lobes lie in front of the occipital lobes, under the parietal and frontal lobes. The top portion of the temporal lobes receive auditory information from the ear. The underside of each temporal lobe plays a crucial role in forming and retrieving memories associated with sounds, especially music. A special area in the lower temporal lobe is responsible for face recognition. Deep within the temporal lobes are other structures which, with the temporal lobes, are involved with memory and sensations of taste, sound, sight, and touch.

Although the lobes may have specific primary responsibilities, none of these zones act in isolation from other areas of the brain. Consider the following example: You hear a selection of music that you remember hearing before and really liking. You have been taking piano lessons for a number of years and can play the piano fairly well. You decide to learn to play this piece yourself. You stop at the music shop and buy a copy of the piano score (sheet music) of this piece. What did your brain do in this scenario? Hearing the music and recognizing the sounds took place in the temporal lobe's auditory cortex. Remembering that you liked this piece involved the temporal lobe, but also structures in the **limbic system**. Your skills in playing the piano involved the motor cortex of the frontal lobes, and deciding to learn to play the piece was part of the "executive function" of the frontal lobes. Going to the music shop used voluntary movement directed by the frontal lobe and coordinated by the cerebellum. Your purchase of the piano score was the action of the frontal lobe, probably using the mathematical skills of the right hemisphere to calculate price, payment, and change. And we have not even taken into consideration your discussion with the clerk at the music store or what went on in your brain when you looked through the music you purchased.

The frontal lobes are located in the forefront of the cerebrum (the forehead area). Possibly because of their dominance in location and thought processes, these frontal lobes often get "first recognition" in discussions of the brain; however, they are not the first zones to develop. In fact, the nerve pathways to the frontal lobes are the last areas to develop.

Now create your own story. Perhaps the music you heard was during an especially exciting, or sad, or romantic scene of a movie you saw. What did your brain do? What if you add to the action a huge bag of warm, buttery popcorn and maybe an air conditioner turned up so high you are shivering? See if you can decide which zones were handling what.

CONNECTIONS

All of these divisions—the two hemispheres, the lobes, and structures within the lobes—are present in a baby's brain at birth. Although a great deal of brain growth and development occurs before birth, much more will take place as the baby and its brain grow after he or she is born.

We have discussed portions of the brain's system that are most easily identifiable. However, within the inner brain there are other systems equally important to the smooth functioning of the brain and the human body as a whole.

2

Structure and Function of Your Brain—Part 2

The body, or some portion of it, is constantly moving, from the prenatal stage and on, as long as there is life. With this movement, the brain is involved. Large areas in the cerebral cortex, and/or the basal ganglia, the cerebellum, the **brain stem**, and the **spinal cord** help initiate and produce this movement. Also, the brain is responsible for controlling the coordination of the body's movements and maintaining body balance. The brain grows and develops as it carries out these processes.

Much of the body's movement is in response to sensory stimuli. Within the cerebral cortex, there are different segments of **sensory cortex** and motor cortex that are devoted to each part of the body. Neurons with related functions are usually arranged in columns. The sensory cortex, located in the parietal lobe, is a band of columns of these neurons that processes the body's physical sensations. The band of neurons that governs voluntary movements is the motor cortex, located in the frontal lobe.

AREAS WITHIN THE INNER BRAIN

Language—a basic foundation of human intelligence—is the primary way we form our thoughts and communicate them to others. It is more than forming words: sometimes language is audible (sounds that we hear) and sometimes language is gestures, such as signing, which is used by many people who are deaf. Language may also be a code—a body of symbols, simple or complex, which must be processed and understood by both sender and receiver in order to have meaning.

As a baby's brain develops, its language of gestures, crying, and babbling, take on meaning as the action satisfies the baby's needs such as food, touching, or comfort. There are distinct types of cries for hunger, anger, and pain. Young babies are very good at mimicking certain facial expressions or hand gestures.

The brains of newborns are primed for language and can recognize some human speech sounds. But many nerve pathways must be developed before they can even begin to make sense of words. This development is largely dependent on their experiences of hearing other people speak. As parents and others talk to a baby, they are activating hearing, social, emotional, and language centers of the baby's brain.

For well over 100 years, scientists have searched for explanations as to how the brain produces and understands language. Before the invention of PET (positron-emission tomography, a brain imaging technique) in the 1980s, scientists investigating language impairments as related to brain

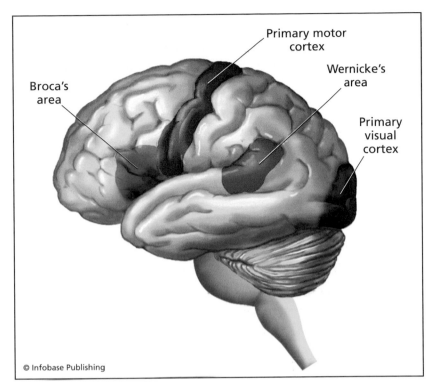

Figure 2.1 Broca's and Wernicke's areas, together with the visual and motor cortices, are responsible for speech and language comprehension.

injuries had to wait until their patients died to confirm their diagnoses. Now, using modern diagnostic methods, researchers are able to determine the primary parts of the brain that specialize in various language operations.

The dominant areas of the brain have been well studied. Two major areas important for language processing are Broca's area and Wernicke's area (Figure 2.1). **Broca's area** is involved in forming words—speech, in other words. It is located in the left frontal lobe, bordering the part of the motor area that controls movement of the face, tongue, mouth, jaw, larynx, and throat.

Wernicke's area is involved in the ability to understand words. It is located in the left back portion of the temporal lobe near the vision, hearing, and touch areas—from which it draws information to recognize and assign meaning to stimuli. For example, when you see a word as you read, the information travels from your visual cortex to Wernicke's area, where the meaning of the word is recognized. The message is trans-

Paul Broca and Carl Wernicke

In the 1860s, Paul Broca, a French surgeon, examined (in autopsies) the brains of people who had lost all or part of their ability to speak. He discovered damage to a particular area in the left frontal lobe. He hypothesized that this damage affected the ability to speak words. His classic case was a patient named Tan. When asked his name, the man answered, "Tan." When asked his address, age, what he wanted to eat, he replied "Tan." Although he understood what he was being asked, he could say only one word. After his death, examination of his brain confirmed injury in the region Broca had predicted.

In the 1870s Carl Wernicke, a German neurologist, discovered a second language area in the left hemisphere of the brain. A person with damage in this area can speak but cannot understand language—neither the language of others nor his own. Sometimes, damage in this area is partial and the injured person loses recognition of nouns and concepts described by nouns. "Cat" or "dog" would be only "animal"—no recognition of difference. However, verbs (run, jump) and adjectives (big, small) were clear.

mitted to Broca's area, which forms the word to be spoken, and then on to the motor cortex for the process of speech.

THE LIMBIC SYSTEM

Some fascinating brain structures lie deep within the brain. A specific group of structures, called the limbic system, forms a ring-like arrangement around the brain stem and links the other parts of the brain with the frontal lobes of the cerebrum/ cerebral cortex. In many references, these terms—*cerebrum* and *cerebral cortex*—are used interchangeably. The cerebral cortex is the outer covering of the cerebrum and contains the concentration of neurons (gray matter). The inside of the cerebrum is predominately a dense network of **axons**, the extensions of nerve cells that serve as the route along which messages travel, sort of like wires looping between telephone poles. Most of the axons are coated with a whitish, insulating cover of **myelin** that keeps the messages moving along swiftly. This area is the "white matter" of the brain. The whole brain is involved in the thinking process, but like any efficient system, certain portions are primarily responsible for specific tasks.

The limbic system is also called the "emotional brain" because it has a lot to do with receiving, interpreting, and controlling emotional experiences. Structures within the limbic system can produce feelings such as fear, anger, pleasure, and sorrow. These are often called the "fight or flight" reactions. Developed during our evolutionary past, this system's job is to guide behavior in a way that may increase the individual's chance of survival.

The limbic system contributes to the retrieval of stored memories, which in turn influence the interpretation of incoming messages. The actions of various parts of the

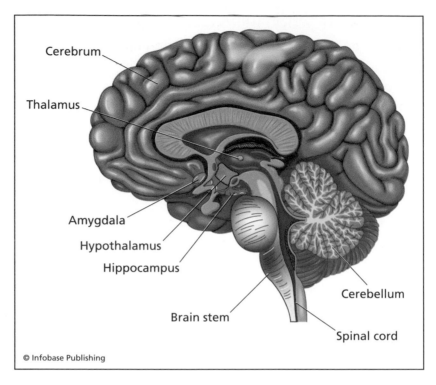

Cerebrum

Thalamus

Amygdala

Hypothalamus

Hippocampus

Brain stem

Cerebellum

Spinal cord

© Infobase Publishing

Figure 2.2 The limbic system is a set of brain structures that work together to produce emotions and feelings. The system, which includes the thalamus, hypothalamus, hippo-campus, and amygdala, also plays a role in learning and memory.

limbic system affect things such as memory, eating disorders, mood fluctuations, and hormones. The parts of the limbic system include the **thalamus**, the **hypothalamus**, the **hippocampus**, and the **amygdala** (Figure 2.2). Each has specific responsibilities, but they all work together to integrate the information coming in from the senses and body organs. There are two of each of these structures, one in each hemisphere.

In the center of the limbic system is the thalamus, which serves as a major clearinghouse or central processing unit for receiving information from the senses (except the sense of smell) and most other information entering the brain. It channels these signals to the appropriate region of the cerebral cortex for interpretation.

Located just below the thalamus, the hypothalamus is the master controller of the **autonomic nervous system**, which governs heart rate, body temperature, appetite and thirst, and the sleep/waking cycle ("body clock"). It also regulates emotions such as anger, pain, pleasure, sexual feelings, and hormone and chemical balances. Eating, sleeping, and sex—all three of these functions depend on nerve cells located in the hypothalamus.

The hippocampus is located inside the temporal lobe and is essential for learning. New information is first coded in this structure as short-term memory, and the hippocampus also processes memories for long-term storage. Memories stored in many parts of brain are indexed here.

The amygdala is an almond-shaped structure located in each of the temporal lobes. It regulates emotions like fear, arousal, and anger. When the amygdala receives stimuli, it determines the "emotional value" of the information received and pairs our responses with experiences. Based on memories of past experiences, the amygdala determines if the particular stimulus is "good" or "bad" and then directs "approach or avoidance" responses to the new experience.

To see how the limbic system works, let's look at an example. It is late at night and you are awakened from sleep by a scratching sound outside your window. You listen intently. For a moment, you hold your breath, then you cautiously peer out the window. It is a windy night and you see the tree by your window. When you recognize that the tree is causing the scratching sound, you immediately relax.

When the scratching sound awakened you, the thalamus received the information of the sound and determined the message needed to be passed on for interpretation. For the interpretation of the possible cause of the sound, the amygdala received the stimuli and determined the emotional value of the sound—is it something to fear or not? Recognizing the source of the sound, aided by the hippocampus's retrieval of information from the memory, the thalamus forwarded information to the cerebral cortex. As you relaxed, the frontal lobes of the cerebral cortex signaled the motor cortex to relax the muscles.

OTHER STRUCTURES OF THE CENTRAL NERVOUS SYSTEM: CEREBELLUM, BRAIN STEM, AND SPINAL CORD

The **cerebellum** is located below the occipital lobes of the cerebrum and just above and behind the brain stem. The name *cerebellum* means "little brain." With its two hemispheres, it looks like a smaller version of the cerebrum, although the folds on its surface are different in appearance from those of the cerebrum. The cerebellum has both gray and white matter, and in an adult weighs about 150 grams (a little more than 5 ounces). It contains nearly 50% of all neurons in the brain, although it constitutes only 10% of total brain volume. One type of neuron in the cerebellum is called the **Purkinje cell**, and there are up to 26 million of them, each of which makes about 200,000 **synapses**. A synapse is the space between nerve cells across which messages are transmitted.

The cerebellum has three functionally distinct regions, each of which constantly receives information from different portions of the brain and spinal cord. The cerebellum compares the movements ordered by the cerebrum with what the body is actually doing: what parts are moving, in what direction, and how fast, and it makes corrections as needed to implement the cerebrum's orders. The cerebellum also ensures balance and coordination by making certain that the muscles of the limbs and trunk work together.

How does all this look in action? Picture the following. There are 20 seconds left in the fourth quarter of your football game, and your team is down by six points. The quarterback fires the ball to you. The brain pathway of this action is:

1 The information about the location of your legs, arms, hands—all your body parts—goes to the cerebellum.
2 Messages from other parts of your brain tell the cerebellum where you need to be.
3 Motor impulses are released that make your muscles move all those necessary body parts. You catch the ball and run for a touchdown.

Consider the parts of the brain that filtered and delivered those messages. The cerebral cortex picked up messages from the visual, auditory, thinking, and memory/emotion centers of your brain as you saw the football, heard the cheers from the crowd, remembered what you are supposed to do, curbed your excitement, and tried to remain calm. The cerebellum received and processed information as to the position of your body and where you needed to be. Then it sent the messages that direct how and where your body parts should move to get to the appropriate location to catch the ball.

The brain stem is located in the lower part of brain and extends from the thalamus to the spinal cord. It is responsible for controlling your breathing, heartbeat, and blood pressure. Scattered throughout the brain stem is a network of nerve cell clusters penetrated by bundles of nerve fibers that give it a net-like appearance. This network is called the **reticular formation**. This system connects centers of the hypothalamus, basal ganglia, cerebellum, and cerebrum. The reticular formation filters incoming sensory impulses, passes on those messages judged to be important and disregards others. This filtering protects the cerebral cortex from continual bombardment of sensory stimulation, allowing it to concentrate on more significant information.

And then there is the spinal cord. The messages between the brain and your body are transmitted to and from the brain

Diagnostic Methods

The recent advances in understanding the brain are due to the development of techniques that allow scientists to directly monitor brain activity.

Electroencephalogram (EEG): The **EEG** records the brain's electrical activity. Electrical signals are detected by a series of electrodes placed on the scalp. These signals are amplified and look like a series of waves when displayed on a monitor or paper chart. The shapes of these waves indicate the brain's activity.

Computerized axial tomography (CAT): The **CAT** scan uses X-ray beams to scan the brain from many different angles. The instrument compares brain densities and produces a detailed cross-section of the brain.

Positron emission tomography (PET): The three-dimensional **PET** scan image indicates metabolic and chemical activity in the brain as well as blood flow, thus showing areas of greatest activity.

through this long cable of nerve fibers encased inside the backbone. The **peripheral nerves** connect with the nerves of the spinal cord to transmit messages to all parts of your body.

THE REFLEX LOOP

Movement is a complex process whether it is reaching for a pencil or catching the pass and running to score a touchdown. Research teams are investigating the neural mechanisms

Magnetic resonance Imaging (MRI): This method is based on the brain's ability to absorb radio waves when surrounded by a magnetic field. Brain structures are clearly visible with this technique, but it does not show anything about brain function.

Functional magnetic resonance imaging (fMRI): The fMRI is a variation of the traditional MRI. Whenever there is increased activity in the brain, blood rushes in to provide extra oxygen and fuel (glucose) for the active brain cells. This brings about small changes in the magnetic field. The fMRI detects areas that are most active.

Magnetoencephalography (MEG): MEG is based on detecting the tiny magnetic pulse emitted in the rapidly changing patterns of brain activity. By combining fMRI (the "where" of brain activity) and MEG (the "when" and "how long" of the activity), researchers can arrive at a much more precise understanding of how the brain works.

underlying voluntary movement, coordination, and balance. There is still much to learn. Catching the ball and running for a touchdown requires the brain to coordinate a number of rapid reactions. As fast as the brain responses are, sometimes they are not fast enough to avoid injury, such as when your hand touches a hot stove or your foot steps on a sharp nail.

Your nervous system has a built-in safety mechanism to minimize the injury from dangers like these. There are short-cuts that order immediate action of body parts in imminent danger through a **reflex loop** that connects directly to and from the spinal cord without waiting for brain action. Your hand immediately jerks back from the stove and your foot flinches from the nail.

CONNECTIONS

Chapters 1 and 2 developed a visual map of the brain and summarized the function of its parts as a guide to understanding how the brain grows. The cerebrum is divided into two hemispheres, which in turn are divided into four lobes—frontal, temporal, parietal, and occipital. Within the frontal lobe is Broca's area, one of the primary areas involved in language processing and production. Situated in the left back portion of the temporal lobe is Wernicke's area, which is involved in the ability to understand language. Located just to the rear of the frontal lobe is the motor cortex. The sensory cortex is in the parietal lobe, which is just behind the motor area of the frontal lobe.

Deep within the brain are a group of structures that make up the limbic system or "emotional brain"—the thalamus, hypothalamus, hippocampus, and amygdala. Located below the occipital lobes is the cerebellum. The brain stem connects the cerebrum and cerebellum to the spinal cord. The information that reaches the brain through the brain stem first goes through the reticular formation.

The central route for transmission of messages between the brain and the body is the spinal cord. Messages to and from the body parts are transmitted to the spinal cord through the peripheral nerves. A built-in safety system from the nerves of the spinal cord to the peripheral nerves is the reflex loop.

The human body works as a team of interrelated systems. The brain is the chief controlling system, which insures smooth functioning of the whole. Now we will turn to how and where these units communicate and function together.

3

The Brain Grows
Communication Leads to Connections

In order for the whole body to act as a unit, all of its parts and systems must be coordinated, which is the task of the nervous system. It is the job of the nerve cells in that system to keep the communication flowing.

The brain's two types of nerve cells are:

◆ Neurons, which receive and transmit messages via electronic impulses

◆ Glial cells (glia), "helper cells" that carry out many support duties that enable the neurons to function and allow communications to flow smoothly.

A great deal of brain development occurs before birth. It has been estimated that by five months into gestation, the fetal brain has nearly 100 billion neurons. The brain continues to produce even more nerve cells after birth and into and beyond child-hood. As it produces nerve cells during its growth phase, the brain will lose or **prune** some of the neurons along the way.

The brain grows in size and importance not only by pro-ducing neurons and glial cells, but also through the large number of connections it makes—more than 10,000 per neu-ron. Stop and consider these numbers: more than 100 billion neurons, each with more than 10,000 connections—that is a trillion connections or more.

Think of making this many Internet connections through wires connected to a trillion Web sites and you can begin to conceptualize the complex mass of neural pathways in your brain alone. You "Google" your brain for the name of your third grade teacher, or the physics formula you need on a test, or a movie now playing at the local theatre. Consider the complex pathways through your neural connections that must be traveled to retrieve that information, and the speed at which your inquiry is answered.

These neural connections are the communication lines to coordinate the many activities of the brain. As specific neural pathways are used repeatedly, that connection is strength-ened. The brain grows as it makes these connections.

NEURONS

The neuron—the key cell of the whole nervous system—has a nucleus and set of genetic instructions in its cell body (Figure 3.1). Extending from that cell body is a long fiber called the axon. Also spreading out from the cell body in a number of directions are shorter, branched extensions called **dendrites**. The cell body and its extensions are each surrounded by a **membrane** that, like a wall, keeps in the **cytoplasm** (a mix of

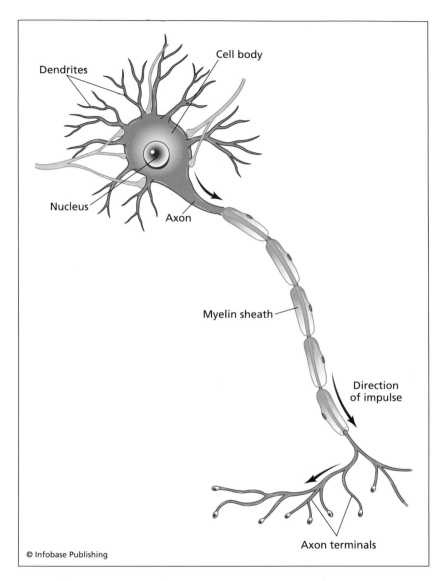

Figure 3.1 The neuron, also known as a nerve cell, transmits chemical and electrical signals throughout the body.

water, proteins, and other materials) and other components of the cell and keeps out unwanted substances.

With its thousands of connections, the neuron needs a well-organized traffic flow of impulses. Dendrites bring electrical signals toward the neuron's cell body, while the axon carries impulses away from the neuron's cell body. Neurons usually have only one axon but may have many dozens of dendrites.

Throughout the system, many of the axons are covered with layers of a fatty substance that form the myelin sheath. In the central nervous system, glial cells called **oligodendrocytes** produce the myelin sheath to insulate the axon. In the peripheral nervous system, glial cells called Schwann cells produce myelin. Impulses travel much faster over myelinated fibers than unmyelinated fibers. For example, think of an electric wire. If the metal wire were not covered with insulation, a short circuit—a disruption of the flow of electricity—would occur whenever the wire touched another wire or stray bits of a conducting material like metal. The myelin sheath around a nerve reminds us, in function, of electrical tape around a wire. Nerve fibers that are myelinated can transmit impulses faster and with much less interference or disruption.

There are three types of neurons:

◆ Sensory neurons receive stimuli and send impulses to the brain and spinal cord.

◆ Motor neurons conduct impulses from the brain or spinal cord to muscles or glands throughout the body.

◆ Interneurons provide connections between sensory and motor neurons (Figure 3.2).

All of these neurons work the same way. When the neuron receives stimuli, those stimuli (or series of stimuli) have to be strong enough to generate an impulse, which is like a tiny electric charge. The neuron sends that impulse out through its axon to other neurons in the target area to be activated.

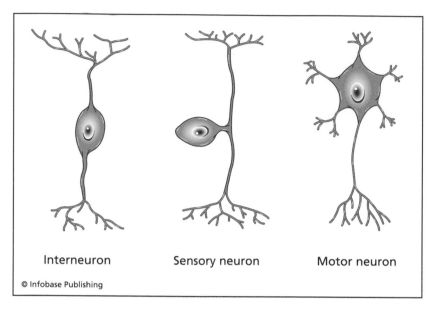

Interneuron   Sensory neuron   Motor neuron

© Infobase Publishing

Figure 3.2 There are three types of neurons in the body. Each type of neuron has the same basic parts but has different functions due to differences in size and shape.

ACTION POTENTIAL

When the neuron is not transmitting an impulse, it is in its "resting" phase. During this period, the inside of the neuron has a net negative charge and the outside has a net positive charge. The neuron continues at this "resting" phase until it receives a stimulus large enough to start a nerve impulse.

The minimum amount of a stimulus that can result in an impulse is called the **threshold**. If the stimulus is weaker than the threshold, there will be no activation of the neuron, and thus no transmitting of the impulse. Once the threshold level is met, the signal triggers what is called the **action potential**.

An action potential is the means by which a neuron sends impulses through the axon toward the next neuron. This process involves electrically charged chemicals called **ions**, which are present in the nervous system. Chemical elements are neutral until they lose or gain electrons. When this occurs, the element is called an ion and is electrically charged—either positive or negative. Those ions important in the nervous system are sodium (Na^+), potassium (K^+), calcium (Ca^{+2}), and chlorine or chloride (Cl^-). Some ions, primarily potassium, can pass through the neuron **cell membrane** fairly easily, but most of the other ions cannot; this is known as **selective permeability**.

The chief means for the other ions to pass into the axon is through an ion channel—a tiny tunnel made of protein, which opens when the threshold level is met. Once threshold is reached, channels that are highly selective for Na^+ open and allow sodium ions to rush inside the cell membrane. This sudden increase of positive charge upsets the electrical balance inside the membrane, generating the action potential by which the positive charge flows forward through the axon. The sudden increase in positive charge from the sodium causes potassium channels to open, allowing K^+ to flow to the outside of the membrane, thus restoring the **resting potential**.

In addition to the selective ion channels, the neuron cell membrane has a sodium–potassium pump system that uses energy to pump Na^+ out of and K^+ into the cell (Figure 3.3). This helps restore and maintain resting potentials. The action potential and resulting current move like waves, generating new action potentials and the subsequent resting potentials, as the impulse is transmitted along the axon.

Once a stimulus has met the threshold level for generating an action potential, the size of all action potentials is always

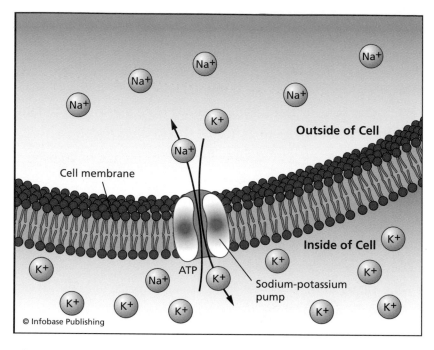

Figure 3.3 A sodium–potassium pump moves sodium ions out of a neuron and potassium ions into the neuron. This action prevents or stops the neuron from firing an electrical signal.

the same. This is true for any neuron. It is called the "all or none" principle. Stimulations of greater intensity will not produce stronger impulses, but rather more impulses per second.

Nerve fibers that are not myelinated conduct impulses over their entire surfaces, resulting in much slower transmission of the signals—maybe only one-half meter per second. Fibers insulated with a myelin sheath transmit impulses rapidly, up to 120 meters per second.

NEUROTRANSMITTERS: THE CHEMICAL MESSENGERS

Impulses travel through the axon until they reach the end of the axon, called the axon terminal. Then there is a gap, a space over which the electrical impulse cannot travel. This space is called the synapse. To get from the end of the axon to the dendrite of the adjacent cell, another means of transport must be used. At the point when the impulses reach the end of the axon they trigger the release of chemicals called **neurotransmitters**. These chemicals are stored in tiny pouches called **vesicles** (Figure 3.4).

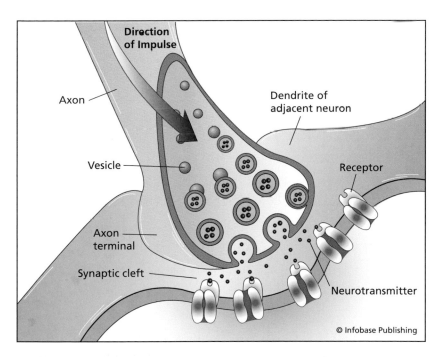

Figure 3.4 In this illustration of a synapse, an electrical impulse causes the release of neurotransmitters from vesicles within the neuron.

The molecules of these neurotransmitters swarm out from their "nesting place" at the end point of the message-sending neuron (**presynaptic neuron**) and diffuse through the fluid in the synapse to the adjacent cell, where they attach themselves to receptor sites on the membrane of the target neuron (**postsynaptic neuron**). The neurotransmitter molecules must fit the receptors like a lock and key to be accepted. New research has shown that some special glial cells called **astrocytes** are also involved in the process.

TYPES OF NEUROTRANSMITTERS

Without transmission across the synapses, messages would go nowhere. There would be no perception, no memory, no singing or speaking, laughing or crying, none of the actions through which you communicate to yourself and to other humans. You would not be able to catch a ball or use your computer. Necessary to performing these all-important transmissions are the neurotransmitters. The nervous system produces many different types of neurotransmitters. Some references indicate over 100 have already been identified. Why so many? Specialization—each kind of neurotransmitter specializes in a specific task. A great deal of current research is trying to find out what the different neurotransmitters are and what they do.

The amino acids **glutamate** and **GABA** (gamma-aminobutyric acid) are the most widespread neurotransmitters in the brain (Figure 3.5). Glutamate tends to be an excitatory neurotransmitter, increasing the likelihood that an action potential will be generated. GABA tends to be an inhibitor, reducing the likelihood of the message being transmitted on to the target or postsynaptic cell. Whether the

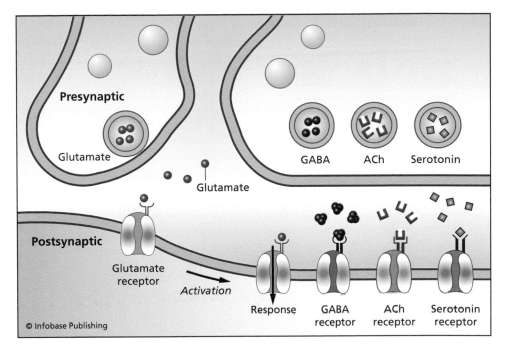

Figure 3.5 Neurotransmitters bind to receptors on the postsynaptic membrane of a neuron. There are many kinds of neurotransmitters, a few of which are noted above.

neurotransmitter acts to excite or to inhibit depends on the receptor or other neurotransmitters influencing the action.

Other chemicals that sometimes effect the action at the synapses are called neuromodulators. These chemicals are less directly involved in the transfer action but act to change or modify the action of glutamate or GABA. Neuromodulators tend to act somewhat slower than glutamate and GABA in responding to the impulse signal, however, they may have a more prolonged effect on the transfer.

Peptides (proteins) can also function as neurotransmitters and are found throughout the body. The best known of those

COMMON NEUROTRANSMITTERS

Listed here are some of the more common neurotransmitters, their functions, and what happens when there is an excess or deficiency of the chemical.

Neurotransmitter	Function(s)	Potential Problem(s)
Glutamate	Important in learning and memory	Excess: Floods brain during a stroke and kills neurons
GABA	Inhibits flow of nerve impulses	Deficiency: Overexcites neurons and can result in epilepsy
Serotonin	Major role in emotions and judgment; also important in controlling sleep, mood, and anxiety; sometimes called the "feel good" chemical	Deficiency: Depression; suicidal behavior; anxiety, impulsive behavior, eating disorders
Dopamine	Regulates mood and movement; involved in memory	Deficiency: Muscle tremors, Parkinson's disease; mental imbalance; lack of attention and concentration; addiction Excess: Hallucinations; schizophrenia; uncontrolled speech and movements, obsessive-compulsive disorder
Norepinephrine	Activated in states of heightened danger; probable role in anxiety, sleep disorders, some mental disorders	Deficiency: Depression

Neurotransmitter	Function(s)	Potential Problem(s)
Acetylcholine	Controls activity in brain areas connected with attention, learning, memory; works at the junction between nerves and muscles, resulting in muscle movement	Deficiency in the brain: May be associated with Alzheimer's disease; delirium, confusion, and memory loss Excess outside the brain: Paralysis of respiratory muscles, which if not treated, can result in death Deficiency outside the brain: Can lead to paralysis and death

peptides active in the brain are the opiates—endorphins and enkephalins. These opiates are triggered by pain and stress and bind to their special receptors to reduce the stress and pain sensations and affect mood as well. Morphine is a drug that mimics peptide neurotransmitters. It has a molecular configuration, or shape, so similar to the peptides that morphine can readily fit into the opiate receptors on the target neuron. While morphine is an effective pain reliever, it is **addictive**. More problematic is that when used in excessive amounts, morphine slows down respiration, sometimes to such a great extent that breathing stops and the person dies.

The monoamines (a class of amines) include serotonin, dopamine, epinephrine, and norepinephrine. The cells that produce these compounds are found mostly in the brain stem, but have axons that extend throughout the brain. These neurotransmitters can produce changes in many brain areas simultaneously and are tremendously important in all of our activities.

Many drugs used in the treatment of psychiatric disorders work by altering the normal activities of these monoamines. For example, Prozac slows the reuptake of serotonin, prolonging serotonin's activity. It is prescribed to treat major depression, obsessive-compulsive disorder, and excessive anxiety. Other drugs such as cocaine, amphetamines, ecstasy, alcohol, and nicotine modify the amounts of serotonin and other monoamines at the synapses, often with detrimental effects. Sometimes, the effects are the death of the nerve endings and permanent depletion of the neurotransmitter. They may also increase heart rate and blood pressure to the extent that there is risk of stroke.

TURNING OFF NEUROTRANSMITTER ACTION

After the natural neurotransmitters have performed their functions in the chemical transport of the signals, the action of the neurotransmitters must be stopped. This deactivation occurs by any of four different mechanisms:

◆ Reuptake—the neurotransmitter molecule is reabsorbed by the axon terminal that released it.

◆ Degradation—molecular disintegration of the neurotransmitter brought about by an enzyme specific to that neurotransmitter.

◆ Diffusion—the neurotransmitter just "drifts away" from the site of the synapse.

◆ Removal—glial cells remove the neurotransmitters from the synapse.

If the "used" neurotransmitter is not deactivated, an excess occurs, which may result in behavioral changes or mental illness.

CONNECTIONS

This chapter has focused on connections and communication. Our brain is made up of billions of specialized cells called neurons. They communicate with each other by receiving and sending messages over tiny fibers—axons and dendrites. When the neurons receive sufficient stimuli to be activated, they transmit their messages by electrical and chemical means to other neurons. The electrical impulses pass through to the end of the axons, where they trigger the release of neurotransmitters into the synapses to transport the message to the target neurons.

The main types of nerve cells are neurons and glia. Projecting from the neuron's cell body are axons over which messages are sent, and multiple dendrites that receive and transport messages to the neuron's cell body. A myelin sheath, which wraps around and insulates the axons, enables the impulses (the electrical component of messages generated by stimuli) to travel much faster through the axon.

Neurotransmitters are chemical compounds released into the synapse—the gap between the end of the axon and the adjacent cell—to transport messages. These messages, now in the form of chemicals, are transported across the synaptic gap from the sending neuron to the receiving or target neuron. The two most widespread of the neurotransmitters are glutamate, which tends to excite, and GABA, which tends to inhibit impulse transmission. In order for chemical neurotransmission to occur properly, the excess neurotransmitters must be removed after they have served their purpose.

4

The Prenatal Period

How our brains develop and grow is an amazing story, one that has its roots in prehistory, the time before written records. If you look at the anatomy of the brain, you can almost trace a good portion of the story of its evolution.

Organisms with only one cell have no nervous system. Multicellular organisms, such as the jellyfish, developed a simple nerve net for communication between the cells. However, a nerve net has no central coordinating component. As cells within these multicellular organisms diversified and became more specialized, the nerve net developed into a nerve cord with nerve fibers—the **notochord**, running the length of the organism's body. The first **chordates** showing evidence of a notochord appeared more than

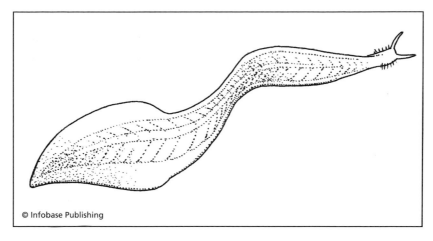

© Infobase Publishing

Figure 4.1 The pikaia lived more than 500 million years ago. It was one of the first animals to have a notochord, which is a primitive form of a spinal cord.

500 million years ago. The example we know of is the pikaia, a soft-bodied animal of the Cambrian Period (Figure 4.1).

As the nerve fibers within the notochord evolved, a cluster of nerve cells or **ganglion** developed in the "head" area. Cerebral ganglia developed in most animals, but only vertebrates developed a head and backbone as we know them. In vertebrates—fish, reptiles, amphibians, birds, mammals—cerebral ganglia developed into primitive brains. These primitive brains were composed of a **forebrain, hindbrain,** and **midbrain,** and a cerebellum for balance and movement.

The forebrain's function varied depending on the species. For fish and amphibians, the very small forebrain area was dedicated completely to the sense of smell. In reptiles, the forebrain developed larger cerebral hemispheres, but it processed only responsive, not "thinking or conscious," reactions. The other basic parts of the primitive brain, the hindbrain and midbrain, evolved into the brain stem. The cerebellum became more complex as movement and balance controlled by the cerebellum became more varied.

As mammals evolved from reptiles, the brain of mammals increased in complexity, adding the limbic system. The early cerebral cortex, which first appeared as a thin "skin" of nerve cells over the cerebral hemispheres of the cerebrum in reptiles, enlarged in mammalian evolution. As more neural connections formed, the cerebrum gradually took on a more dominant role in the organism—so much so that the cerebral cortex added more and more convolutions, loops, and folds, permitting the increasing brain growth to fit within the tight confines of the skull. With the development of the cerebral cortex/cerebrum came the ability to receive and process more information.

The early human brain is estimated to have weighed less than a pound. As *Homo habilis* made tools, his brain grew. A million years ago, *Homo erectus* discovered the use of fire and hunting and his brain size doubled. Our brains, especially the frontal lobes, have expanded by some 40% as compared with these early ancestors.

This expansion of the brain eventually pushed the forehead outward from the flat forehead shape of the earlier human ancestors. The expanded brain, especially the frontal lobes, is responsible for reshaping the head into the modern skull of humans today. Our brains have grown to weigh about three pounds. The specific cerebral functions of our brains in those frontal lobes—the thinking, planning, organizing, and communicating—are unique to humans (*Homo sapiens*).

The brain's growth of nerve cells and increasing connections is dynamic, constantly shaping and reshaping as influenced by our genes, our environment, and our choices. It is this extent to which we are able to think and make choices that "make us human."

EARLY BRAIN GROWTH AND DEVELOPMENT

Until recently, research scientists studied prenatal brain growth in two main ways—either by examining fetuses that did not survive until birth or through studies of animals. A number of different animals have been used—roundworm, fruit fly, frog, zebra fish, mouse, rat, chicken, cat, and particularly monkeys because the monkey brain most resembles those of people.

With today's **imaging technology,** we can study the brain of a fetus in the womb. The use of magnetic resonance imaging (MRI) for evaluating possible fetal complications allows the actual brain action and development to be examined. There is no convincing evidence that MRI poses a risk to the fetus. However, there is some question about having MRI procedures during the first trimester until more studies confirm its safety for a fetus during that early stage of development.

One of our questions was "Where did the brain come from?" It is part of the genetic blueprint of all organisms from their beginning. Your human brain has been growing since a single sheet of cells began to divide, producing neurons, at about six weeks after you were conceived. Most of the early cell divisions occurred on the inside surface of the neural tube.

In prenatal development, the first sign of the developing nervous system in the fetus is a thickening cell mass called the **neural plate**. A crease or fold appears that forms a

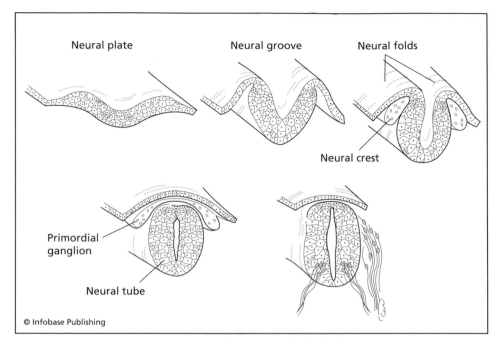

Neural plate   Neural groove   Neural folds

Neural crest

Primordial ganglion

Neural tube

© Infobase Publishing

Figure 4.2 A key point in the development of the human nervous system is the formation of the neural plate. The neural plate folds to create the neural tube, which over the course of many weeks will form the brain and the rest of the nervous system.

"trench" in this neural plate. This fold or trench is the **neural groove**, which runs the length of the neural plate, dividing it into right and left halves. These two halves develop into the right and left hemispheres—or right and left brain.

By about the third or fourth week from conception, a **neural tube** is formed when the edges of the neural groove meet (Figure 4.2). As these edges arch over and fuse, closure of the neural tube occurs. If closure is incomplete, serious problems can occur, such as spina bifida, which can sometimes be corrected by surgery. When the closure of the neural tube is complete, the front part of this structure develops into the primitive brain. Slight swellings represent its three major areas—the forebrain, midbrain, and hindbrain. The remainder of the neural tube develops into the spinal cord. At this state of development, the human embryo is about one-tenth of an inch long.

As the embryo enters the second month of its development, the pace of cell growth increases. Changes occur in these three primitive brain structures—forebrain, midbrain, and hindbrain—which resemble the brain of the early vertebrates. In the front portion of the neural tube, primitive brain cavities develop. These vacant areas become fluid-filled spaces known as the ventricles. The cerebrospinal fluid (CSF) produced in the ventricles will nourish the nerve cells and act as a cushion to protect the brain and spinal cord.

CELLULAR DIFFERENTIATION

Deep inside the brain, along the surface of the ventricles in the neural tube, are born the brain's cells—the neurons and glial cells. The primitive brain cells begin to migrate outward, traveling along particular pathways to reach their preprogrammed destinations. It is not clear exactly how the genetic "blueprints" control where the cells go, but we do know that the cerebral cortex is built in layers. In a process that continues for most of the gestation period, the cerebral cortex builds itself from the inside layer first, then layer by layer outward to its sixth layer.

This complex process of cell multiplication and migration is driven and controlled by a number of different chemical substances that the body itself supplies. Some of the primitive cells become neurons and some become glial cells. Neurons transmit the electrical impulses that carry out the primary communications of the brain—the thinking, interpreting, and controlling actions of the brain. Glial cells are the support cells, providing structural support, nutrition, insulation, and, as has been recently discovered, they also provide assistance at synapses. When the primitive migrating neurons reach their final positions, they begin to develop extensions to their cell bodies. The neuron "sprouts" axons and dendrites and is able to send and receive messages across a synapse.

THE DEVELOPING FETAL BRAIN

At this point, the prenatal brain is changing rapidly (Figure 4.3). The neurons continue to grow tremendously, with peak growth occurring in the fourth and fifth months of pregnancy. The growth spurt then tapers off, but growing still continues, although not quite as fast. By the sixth or seventh month, 70% of the brain's neurons are located in the cerebral cortex (outer layer of the brain).

For the first four or five months of development, the surface of the fetal brain was quite smooth. But in the latter part of the seventh month, much of the fetal skull has begun to harden as the cartilage throughout the embryo turns to bone. This limits the amount of space available for the brain to grow outward. As a result, the surface of the brain "folds in on itself" repeatedly, becoming quite wrinkled. These folds, provide increased surface area to allow for the vast number of neurons that have formed. During the brain's peak growth stage in the last three months of pregnancy, it is estimated that 250,000 neurons are formed every minute.

Growth occurs all through gestation, but during some periods the brain's growth is more rapid than others. Periods of

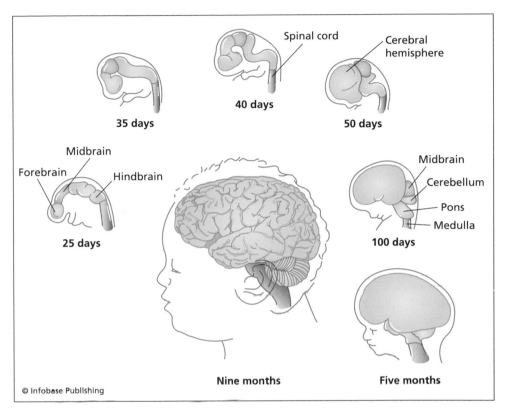

Figure 4.3 This illustration depicts the development of the human brain while inside the mother's womb.

"overproduction" of neurons are followed by some "paring back" or pruning to form a more stable system. It is estimated that the number of neurons at birth surpasses 100 billion, and the number of connections within the brain itself is as many as 75 trillion.

MYELINATION AND PLASTICITY

Myelination is the process by which the fatty substance myelin wraps around the axons (Figure 4.4). This insulation

Developmental Risks

With millions of cells multiplying each day, much can potentially go wrong. If certain drugs and substances (for example, alcohol, tobacco, and illegal drugs) are ingested during pregnancy, they increase the risk that developmental mistakes will happen. Alcohol in the mother's bloodstream passes into the placenta easily and can interfere with brain development. Smoking, or use of any form of tobacco, affects the fetus's physical development, including brain development. Drugs such as cocaine, heroin, and marijuana can have a devastating effect on fetal development. Even some over-the-counter medications and dietary supplements could potentially cause problems.

There are public health programs designed to inform people of these risks, with the anticipation that awareness of these concerns will lower the risk of a child being born with mental retardation or other conditions. Health classes in schools also typically include this information. The whole complex process of brain development is amazing. The more that potential parents know about it, the better care they can take of themselves, and the better chance the fetus has to develop without complications.

is critical for the speed and efficiency of the transmission of impulses. Myelin acts as insulation and protects crucial neural connections. The process of myelination begins for the fetus in about the eighth month and continues on into childhood, occurring when and where it is needed. The "when" and "where" are determined by the developing stages of the emerging organism—baby, child, teen, or young adult. This

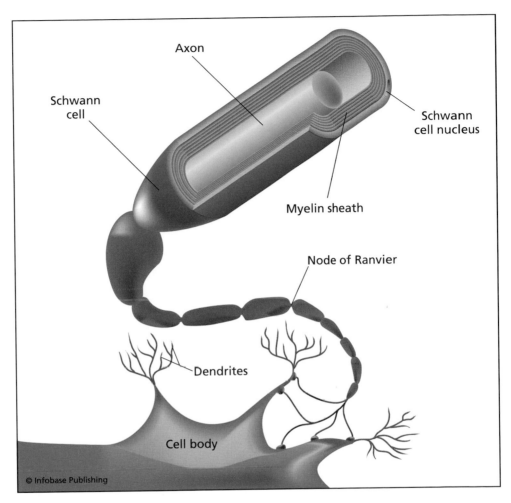

Figure 4.4 **Layers of myelin are wrapped around the axon of a neuron. In the peripheral nervous system, the myelin is manufactured by a specialized cell known as a Schwann cell. In the central nervous system, oligodendrocytes manufacture myelin.**

myelination process will occur at different times in different parts of the brain. Research is now showing that even in adults myelination occurs to repair axons' myelin sheaths.

In general, the axons of neurons in the sensory and motor areas are myelinated first, protecting these areas before birth. Myelination of axons involved with additional coordination skills occurs later and will enable the baby to better control arm and leg movements, usually at about six to nine months of age.

Plasticity of the brain is one of its key features from the development of the fetal brain to the child's brain and beyond. Plasticity refers to the brain's ability to be molded or reshaped, changing as circumstances require. The features of the brain's development are a combination of the preprogrammed instructions encoded in genes and exposure to the environment, both in the womb and after birth. Genes govern the type of brain cell produced, its location, function, and the type of neurotransmitters to which it will respond. Throughout life, environmental, genetic, and choice factors interact in brain development. Whether a particular neuron will develop further or go unused and wither away depends on external stimulation—everything from sight to sound to stress—as expressed by the phrase "use it or lose it."

CONNECTIONS

Components of the earliest brains in vertebrates were the cerebellum, hindbrain, midbrain, and forebrain. In reptiles, the hindbrain and midbrain evolved into the brain stem. In the early species, the cerebellum, serving as the "major brain," controlled balance and movement. In the evolution of mammals, the cerebral hemispheres became larger and the cerebrum became dominant. As the cerebral cortex added more and more nerve cells, this covering of the cerebrum had to "crunch up," folding and twisting in order to fit within the limited space of the skull.

In the human prenatal phase, the brain goes through and moves far beyond the stages of development of earlier species. Neurons and glial cells are formed deep within the brain and migrate to their genetically determined destinations. Cell differentiation and myelination occur and glimpses of the brain's plasticity are evident.

Now, we turn to the development of the brain as the child progresses through the first five years (Chapter 5), then through the school years (Chapter 6), and into adolescence (Chapter 7).

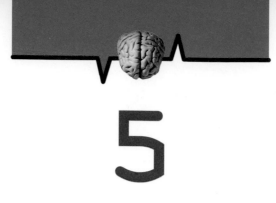

5

The First
Five Years

When the human baby is born, making its first appearance outside the protective environment of the womb, its brain is a fragile substance encased within an armor of bone and cartilage. Already partitioned into sections designated for specific functions, this little brain—weighing less than a pound—directs the usual howling, kicking, and gasping for breath that accompanies this moment of arrival.

In the first hours and days after birth, the newborn's **reflexes**, such as "jerking" when startled, yawning, coughing, and sneezing, are controlled by the brain stem and other structures below the cortical layer. The brain stem is located beside the cerebellum connecting the spinal cord to the cerebral hemispheres.

MAJOR SENSES PRESENT AT BIRTH

What we have discussed about the brain's components and how they communicate, we now apply to brain growth during the first five years of a child's life. As we focus on the major senses and the influence of the inner brain, we see how these early years set the stage for important future brain growth and development.

Touch

Touch is the first sense to emerge in the newborn. Although the sense of touch is by no means fully developed at birth, newborns can "feel" a lot better than they see, hear, or even taste or smell. Touch is one of a newborn's most advanced and better developed senses.

These sensory pathways develop to some extent even before birth. Within the womb, the fetus was enveloped by fluid and in contact with the lining and muscles of the womb. (There are some indications that smell and taste may also be involved in this prenatal interaction.) The "registering" of these sensations in the womb is basically with the primordial brain stem as opposed to cognitive recognition by the cerebrum. The nerve pathways are not, at this point, sufficiently developed to transmit messages to the cerebrum.

Research has shown the importance of continued physical contact and emotional attachment of the baby during the days, weeks, and months after birth. Some researchers think that babies develop the foundations of their stress response system during this early development. Specific evidence of babies adopted from Romanian orphanages, where touching and cuddling were limited, found these children had

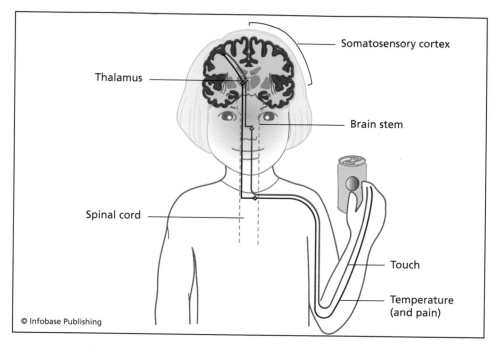

Figure 5.1 Touch sensations move up the spinal cord toward the brain, then are relayed by the thalamus to the somatosensory cortex.

difficulty forming emotional attachments even within later warm and supportive environments. This is consistent with other studies involving rats and monkeys, which show that neglectful care early in life and lack of parental support when an infant is distressed has a powerful influence on the ways their stress response systems develop.

In considering the nerve pathways, these sensations of touch are initially simple reflex reactions involving only sensory neurons and motor circuits within the spinal cord. Later, sensory fibers reach the brain stem. From the brain stem the sensations are relayed to the thalamus in the inner brain (Figure 5.1). The axons of the thalamus form synapses to a

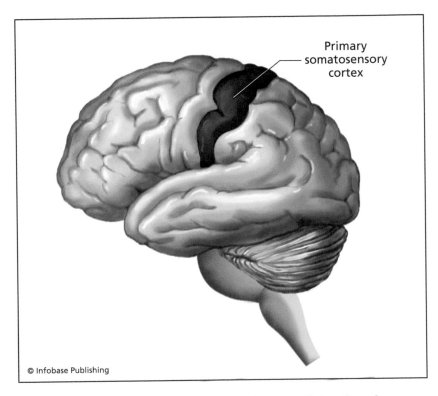

Primary
somatosensory
cortex

© Infobase Publishing

Figure 5.2 The somatosensory cortex consists of regions that are responsible for touch sensation in different parts of the body.

portion of the somatosensory cortex located in the parietal lobes (Figure 5.2).

The mouth is the first region to become sensitive. Babies explore everything with their mouths, no matter how yucky or dangerous. Touch sensitivity develops in a head-to-toe sequence. That is, sensitivity develops around facial areas first and foot areas last. Newborn girls seem to be more sensitive to touch than newborn boys, and this difference persists on throughout life.

Smell

The baby's sense of smell is quite sensitive and one of the more advanced abilities at birth. Young babies can recognize their mothers' scent. Newborns react to odors—to unpleasant odors by crying or turning away, to pleasant odors by sucking motions or turning their faces toward the odor source. This smell or olfactory sensitivity appears to increase steadily over the first few weeks. Consistent differentiation between "good" or "bad" odors (as distinguished from what appears to be reflexive response) begins around age three. Interestingly, female babies seem to be more responsive to odors than male babies, a sensitivity that seems consistent among females of all ages.

Taste

When it comes to taste, newborns can tell the difference between many different flavors, but consistently want only sweet tastes. This preference continues through early child-hood. To sour and bitter tastes, newborns wrinkle their noses, purse their lips, drool or salivate, and generally give an angry reaction. To salt, they are normally indifferent, seeming not to taste it at all.

Although research detects a definite preference in tastes, babies do not consciously choose certain tastes. When you consciously choose something, you use the cerebral cortex, the thinking part of your brain. Where babies are concerned, reflex circuits, which come from the brain stem alone, can control these responses to taste. Since the receptors for taste and touch are very close to each other in the mouth and tongue, and we know touch pathways to the brain develop very early, it is possible that taste may form conscious pathways early.

Whether parents like it or not, children continue what seems to be a "nature-directed" preference to sweetened rather than unsweetened foods throughout their preschool years. Of course, as they get older, experience does play a role. By school age and older, liking or not liking sweets is a matter of conscious choice, but it is also influenced by what neurotransmitters are released when they eat sweets.

Although there is no indication that young children have any preference for fatty substances, it should be noted that infants and toddlers need a larger proportion of total fat in their diet than do older children and adults. Fats are crucial for myelination of axons and for growth and wiring of neurons.

Hearing

By birth, babies have had about twelve weeks of listening experiences in the womb. As newborns, they seem to have memories of their prenatal auditory experiences. Newborns have a narrow range of hearing and in order to hear, need louder sounds than do adults. Newborns are able to hear words in normal conversational tones, but probably not faint whispers. The need for louder sounds decreases as the auditory fibers from the thalamus to the auditory cortex in the temporal lobe continue to develop. Toddlers and pre-school age children hear better than babies, needing only about tenfold (10dB) louder sounds than adults. Hearing gradually improves until puberty, when it is actually more sensitive than adults—that is, until listening to loud music begins to take its toll.

Common Sound Levels

The decibel (dB) is a unit used to express the intensity of a sound wave. By convention, zero decibels ("0" dB) is designated as the threshold of human hearing; that is, the lowest level of sound "loudness" (volume, amplitude of sound waves) that human hearing can detect. Every 10 decibel (10 dB) increase is 10 times louder. An increase of 20 decibels is 10^2 or 100 times louder. Normal conversation is held at about 60 decibels (60 dB). Babies, even newborns, can hear normal conversations, but it is not until they are older that their hearing is as acute as adults'.

Common Sound Levels

Decibels (dB)	Type of Sound
0	Threshold for human hearing
20	Faint whisper
40	Average home noise
60	Normal conversation
80	Heavy traffic; ringing telephone
100	Subway train, power mower
120	Loud thunder
140	Jet plane 100 feet overhead (this level can cause pain and damage)

Source: Lise Eliot. *What's Going On in There?* (New York: Bantam Books, 1999): p. 230.

Sight

What the human baby can see at birth is probably only fuzzy objects. At first, vision focuses best from about a foot away, because the retinal structures from the eyes and the optic nerves are underdeveloped. Some brain growth is genetic and some is based on experiences—sight is one of those senses in which development is highly dependent on experience. For this reason, we will consider the sense of sight as an example of how the brain grows through the development of this sense.

At birth, the baby will be able to see clearly only about eight inches' distance, and the details of faces and objects will be a blur. However, sight begins developing right away and by six months of age, all of the baby's primary visual abilities will have emerged. The brain devotes more of its territory to vision than to all the other senses combined.

Vision begins in the eye when light strikes **photoreceptors** located in the retina (Figure 5.3). Photoreceptors are specialized nerve cells that can capture a single light particle, called a **photon**, and convert its energy into a chemical reaction. This reaction in turn produces an electrical signal that begins the process of neural transmission or signals. These signals divide onto different pathways. One pathway goes to the brain stem, where visual information is used to control eye movements and reflexes. This pathway operates at an entirely subconscious level and is not responsible for what we commonly think of as "seeing."

The other pathway projects signals to the visual area of the thalamus, the part of the inner brain that "directs traffic." The thalamus sends the visual information via impulses to a special area in the occipital lobe of the cerebral cortex, where it goes through a number of steps to process these signals into

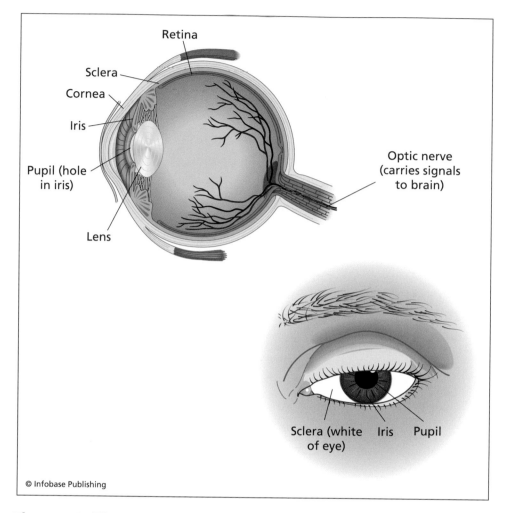

Retina

Sclera

Cornea

Iris

Pupil (hole in iris)

Lens

Optic nerve (carries signals to brain)

Sclera (white of eye)   Iris   Pupil

© Infobase Publishing

Figure 5.3 The eye converts light energy into electrical signals that are carried by the optic nerve to the brain.

what we see. For example, if a blue bike speeds by, we do not notice that our brain has separately processed the shape, color, location, and direction of motion of that bike. We see a shape we recognize as a bike, its color is blue, and it is moving. Many areas of the brain provided input in order for us to "see" that bike.

Although we associate visual pathways with the occipital lobe, there are many other regions in the brain that process certain aspects of visual information. Researchers have identified 32 areas devoted to vision in each hemisphere of the brain. Think about how many different things you see in a minute, let alone in a whole day, and how all these areas of your brain are involved in each one.

Neurobiologists have determined that visual development occurs in two phases. The first is controlled by genes (nature), which establish an overall general "wiring." This is the stage of the baby at birth. The second phase is directed by experience (nurture) or what the baby sees in those first days, weeks, and months after birth. The synapses are formed and strengthened by use; those nerve pathways that are not used wither and die.

For sight, there seems to be a critical time period in which visual experience must occur. The synapses that initially form with the baby's first experiences remain plastic and subject to modification by experience as long the synapses are in their **refinement phase**. The connection between the eye and the occipital lobe must be established in order for sight to be developed in that eye. But just how long the critical time period is for humans remains a question.

BRAIN GROWTH THROUGH ACTIONS AND EXPERIENCES

The brain grows through what it does. Like the CEO (chief executive officer) of any business, or the quarterback of a football team, the brain has to obtain information as to what is going on around it. The sensory system we have been concentrating on supplies the brain with this information. The neurons grow because, as they obtain these sensory signals, they make more connections to process the information.

In order to "juggle" all the information coming into it, the brain has a filtering system, the reticular formation, that lets some of the messages through and blocks or redirects others. In this way, the brain does not get overwhelmed with so many simultaneous messages.

In sensory systems, the information travels primarily in one direction—from the outside world to the brain. But for those messages that get through the filtering system, the brain must respond or react in some way. Most of these responses involve movement: some movements require conscious decisions, while others are unconscious or reflexive.

The brain stem is involved in the control of the most basic body functions, such as heartbeat, blood pressure, digestion, and breathing. You do not have to use the "thinking" part of your brain to consciously direct these activities. The autonomic nervous system, working through reflexes and the brain stem, takes care of the internal monitoring and control of the body organs.

MOVEMENT AND REFLEXES

When it is necessary for the body to react quickly to avoid danger or injury, immediate action is needed. You quickly jerk your hand away from the hot stove before your thinking brain recognizes the danger or feels the pain. The sensory nerves relay these danger messages directly to the spinal cord, where the motor neurons immediately activate the nec-

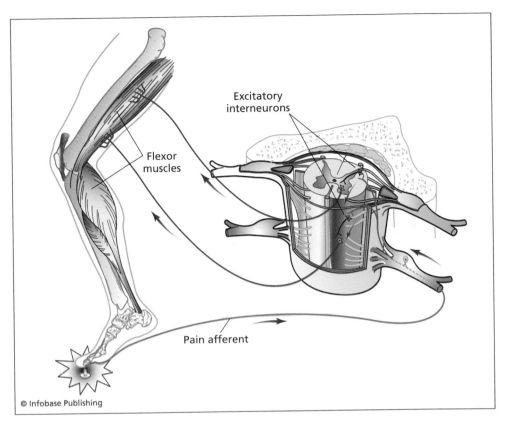

Excitatory
interneurons

Flexor
muscles

Pain afferent

© Infobase Publishing

Figure 5.4 The flexor reflex occurs after pain receptors in the skin are triggered (such as after stepping on a tack, as illustrated above). Sensory neurons then transmit the pain signal directly to the spinal cord. The signal is then relayed to the muscles, which contract to withdraw the injured limb from the source of pain.

essary muscle movements. These are reflexes and this route is called the reflex loop (Figure 5.4). In a second pathway, messages travel to the cerebral cortex, where the brain recognizes the pain or danger and the action taken. This is an efficient way for the systems to operate.

Motor areas in the cerebral cortex, located in the back half of the frontal lobes, direct conscious, or voluntary, movement. As in other systems, signals from the left side of the brain cross over to the right side of the body and vice versa. Even a simple movement requires complex neural processing. And in all of these actions, the brain is growing. More complex movements, like walking, running to catch a football, and playing the violin, are complicated. Keeping all of these movements coordinated is the job of the cerebellum.

Located at the back of the brain, the cerebellum receives messages from the motor cortex indicating what kind of movement is being attempted. Then, it gets signals from the senses as to what movement is actually happening. By comparing all this information, it directs any necessary corrections. The cerebellum is also involved in the storage of some motor skills that come from practice and repetition, like riding a bike or playing the piano. All of this coordination and implementation of movement is so important that even though the cerebellum accounts for only about 10% of the brain's volume, it contains more than half of the neurons in the brain.

At first, a baby's movements are jerky reflexes, and then they become more controlled and intentional. At about nine months old, the baby is crawling, and by a year or so, walking. Motor pathways develop, the cerebellum forms new neurons, myelinations occur, and the toddler learns motor skills. These neural pathways are repeated and strengthened and, over time, become permanent.

In the first five years, the brain grows and neural connections increase through the development and use of the senses and movements. But the picture of brain growth does not end there.

THE INFLUENCE OF THE INNER BRAIN

Deep within the cerebral hemispheres, the limbic system of the brain shapes the social and emotional growth of the child. The emotional skills of the child—and adults, too—are governed by a large set of neural structures called the limbic system, which includes the amygdala and the hypothalamus. Situated between the cerebral cortex and the brain stem, the limbic system influences communication, perception, decision-making, and even a baby's smile.

If the amygdala receives stimuli that it interprets to represent a threat, it activates the hypothalamus, triggering the release of hormones that set into motion a "fight or flight" response. Emotion is not the only task of the limbic system. Many of these structures play a crucial role in memory

The Strange Case of Phineas Gage

In 1848, an industrious, friendly, honest young railroad foreman named Phineas Gage was caught in an explosion, which sent a 13-pound iron rod tearing through his left cheek, behind his left eye. It went through his left frontal lobe and out his skull. He recovered physically from the injury, but his behavior was drastically changed. Phineas seemed like a completely different person. He was no longer a good worker; he lied, stole, and cursed. Years later, when his preserved skull was examined using modern imaging techniques, it was determined that the rod had gone through the prefrontal cortex. Subsequently, it was discovered that damage to the prefrontal cortex impairs a person's ability for behavior control.

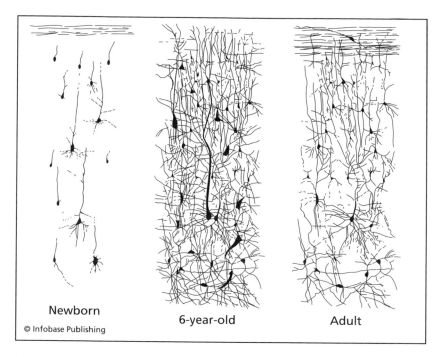

Newborn

6-year-old

Adult

© Infobase Publishing

Figure 6.2 By about age six, neuron connections are at maximum density. In the following years, the number of connections decreases as a result of pruning.

learned at different ages for different children, depending on their individual experiences.

PRIME TIME FOR LANGUAGE DEVELOPMENT

Language development, especially spoken language, is greatly affected by the age of the learner. One's native language, and additional languages as well, are more easily learned when the individual is young. The period for optimal learning for languages does seem to close, slowly, around puberty. Languages can be learned later, but it is usually harder to detect sound differences in pronunciation. The "closing of the door" is not true of vocabulary: the brain takes in new words and language forms well beyond childhood. It continually adds new words to those basic languages learned in earlier years.

Language systems situated further back in the brain (Wernicke's and Broca's areas) undergo a rapid growth spurt around the ages of 11 to 15. Then, the growth spurt

Einstein's Brain

Nobel Prize–winning physicist Albert Einstein died in 1955. During the autopsy, pathologist Thomas Harvey removed Einstein's brain, put it in a jar of formaldehyde, and took it home with him. The rest of Einstein's body was cremated. Dr. Harvey gave bits of the famous brain to researchers, but he kept most of it himself for over 40 years.

Examinations of Einstein's brain found that it weighed somewhat less than the average adult male, that the thickness of the prefrontal cortex was thinner, and that the density of neurons was greater when measured up against other brains researchers compared with it. Another study found that Einstein's brain was 15% wider in the parietal region, an area of the brain that is important for spatial reasoning and mathematical abilities. The researcher who conducted this study, Sandra Witelson, Ph.D., of the Department of Neuropsychology, at McMaster University, said, "We held Einstein's brain in our hands and realized that this is the organ that was responsible for changing our perceptions of the universe, and we were in awe."

drastically shuts off. This is consistent with what teachers and others thought to be the most efficient age to learn new languages.

The biggest surprise is how much tissue the brain loses in the teen years: it is estimated that up to 50% of brain tissue in the deep motor nuclei is lost. These systems control motor skills such as writing, playing sports, or learning to play the piano. This loss moves like a wildfire into the frontal lobes in late teens.

Although it is harder to learn a language when you are older, that does not mean it is impossible. You can learn new languages at older ages; however, you may not speak a new language with the same "natural accent" as one who learns the language at a younger age. We know the brain is flexible. It can learn new words along with a lot of other new things, and it would be unwise to underestimate what the brain can do. Albert Einstein, who they say did not talk until he was three years old, did amazing things with his brain. The brain keeps forming new connections and learning takes place throughout our lives.

NEURON PRUNING

Your brain weighs between 1,300 and 1,400 grams, or about 3 pounds. It is estimated to contain approximately 100 billion neurons with 150 trillion to 240 trillion synapses in the cerebral cortex.

The process of pruning occurs even before birth, but the prenatal growth of neurons is tremendously greater than the pruning. Perhaps the brain produces an excess of nerve cells, thus meeting the potential needs of the growing organism. After birth, the overproduction of neurons continues and is followed by pruning of those neurons not needed or not activated.

The two processes—growth and pruning—continue throughout life, but the relative balance of the processes changes. In the early years, the growth of neurons far outpaces the pruning. From age 4 or 5 until roughly the age of 10, the growth and formation of new connections are balanced by the elimination of the ones that are not used. A somewhat explosive increase in growth occurs in the latter part of this time period, up to the ages of 11 to 15. With puberty, the balance shifts and the pruning of connections exceeds the formation of new ones.

Pruning is not "bad" unless, of course, it occurs in an area you later want to use. You can think of pruning as a means of traffic control. The excess nerve cells that are not in use die off. It is estimated that we lose about one neuron per second in the **neocortex**, which is the largest part of the cerebral cortex. This process shapes the brain and allows it to respond more efficiently in the direction that our use of neural networks has indicated.

Pruning is central to our understanding the brain, its growth, and what we mean by its plasticity. When we are born, our brain develops partly because of genetic instructions (nature) and partly because of our experiences and exposure to the outside world (nurture). Experiences cause our neural networks, our synapses, to grow stronger. The absence of experiences results in the pruning or withering of the related neural networks no longer used. These processes are how the brain continues to grow throughout life.

The brain of an adult can "rewire" itself, that is, form new connections, throughout life into old age. However, it is in the early through late teen years that this process—rewiring and forming new connections—is most pronounced. The brain undergoes shaping much like pruning a tree determines the shape of that tree. Much of what is pruned is influenced by one's experiences and one's choices.

Why some stages of development are extremely time-sensitive, such as sight, and others develop over much longer times, we do not yet know. Researchers believe that the "use it or lose it" principle applies to all aspects of brain development, everything from hearing and movement to thinking and feeling.

CONNECTIONS

The brain continues to grow and develop much longer than researchers previously thought. Brain imaging scans indicate faster growth just before puberty, but at the onset of puberty there is a sharp decline in the fast growth and the rate of pruning increases. For the 6- to about 12-year olds, the highest rates of brain growth are in the areas specializing in language and associative thinking, the ability to "put things together," see relationships, and make connections. These years are the prime time for establishing learning pathways, especially for languages. Times for learning other skills are not so clear-cut, and learning many other skills is a lifelong process.

Patterns sown in the earlier years shape much of the teenage years. Adolescent brain growth and development is a combination of challenges and opportunities. We will look into these exciting, sometimes turbulent times in the next chapter.

7

The Teen Brain

All of the brain pathways that you use will be reinforced each time you use them. For example, if you wanted to play the piano or violin, the nerve pathways you learn in each practice session get stronger as they are used and thus reinforced. The same is true if you draw, do math problems, write essays, or totally "veg out." What you use, you are more likely to retain and improve in, while the nerve pathways and connections you do not use are more likely to wither away and die.

That is not to say you will never play football or play the piano or write if you do not learn to do so before adolescence. It just means that skills you give up on now will not be as easy to recapture later. And you may not reach the level of proficiency you would have reached had you continued to use those pathways while you are still young.

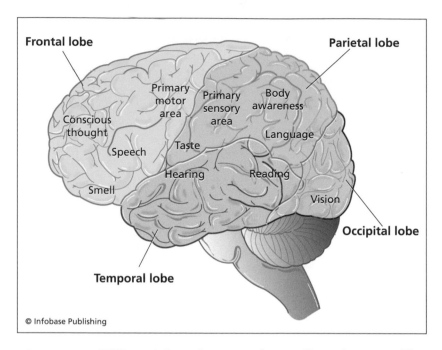

Frontal lobe

Parietal lobe

Primary motor area

Primary sensory area

Body awareness

Conscious thought

Language

Speech

Taste

Hearing

Reading

Smell

Vision

Occipital lobe

Temporal lobe

© Infobase Publishing

Figure 7.1 **Different functions can be attributed to specific areas of the brain. For example, vision is primarily associated with the occipital lobe, while speech can be pinpointed to the frontal lobe.**

Pruning in the brain is like clearing a space in your room: the brain has to do some pruning of the less used neural networks in order to strengthen those neural connections you do use. This clears the "clutter" and enables the brain to work more efficiently. You cannot predict or determine all your future activities, but you do want to keep your options open.

The frontal lobe of the brain is where the thinking processes go on—reasoning, problem solving, making decisions, and carrying them out (Figure 7.1). All that tremendous growth during the pre-puberty years gave the brain enormous potential and the capacity to be skilled in many different areas. Then, at the onset of puberty, the pruning-down phase started. There is a substantial loss in gray matter in the frontal lobes from the mid-teens through the mid-twenties.

Instead of being scary, pruning is challenging. At this age, you have some say in what happens. Those nerve cells and connections that are used will survive and grow stronger, so each person can help determine what he or she chooses to keep.

Protect Your Brain

Because the adolescent years are such a critical time for brain growth and development, it is important to protect the brain from harm and to nurture its learning capabilities. One area of particular concern during these teen years is the use of alcohol and illegal drugs, which have the potential to do irreparable harm to the brain.

Dr. Jay Giedd, a neuroscientist at the National Institute of Mental Health and one of the leading researchers in studying the growth and change in the adolescent brain, said during a television interview, "It's a particularly cruel irony of nature . . . that right at this time when the brain is most vulnerable is also the time when teens are most likely to experiment with drugs or alcohol." These substances could end up influencing or harming the brain for a long time, particularly in the areas of learning and memory. As Dr. Giedd cautioned, "It may not just be affecting their brains for that night or even for that weekend, but for the next 80 years of their lives." Taking care of yourself with good health habits and staying away from substance abuse are crucial during these years.

It is important to understand why adolescence is a critical time for brain growth. In this period, significant intellectual processes are appearing. The adolescent is moving from concrete thinking, which dominated thought patterns when he or she was younger, to abstract thinking and the beginnings of awareness of his or her own thought processes. Emerging also is the ability to do problem solving and think critically—that is, evaluate, analyze, plan, and control impulses. These skills apply whether your future leads to analyzing a car engine, preparing a legal brief, designing a rocket launch, or laying a house foundation.

MAKING MEMORIES

Research has shown that there are different forms of memory. One kind is our conscious recall of facts, people, places, and events, which is called **declarative memory**. This kind of memory passes through the hippocampus before it is recorded in the cerebral cortex. The other primary kind of memory, **nondeclarative memory**, is a recall, without conscious effort, of things like various skills, habits, or procedural memory—how we do things.

We also have **sensory memory**, which holds information from our eyes, ears, and other senses for a short time before that information is incorporated into a declarative or nondeclarative memory system. The input from the amygdala generates **emotional memory**, which can color or influence all forms of memory with positive or negative overtones.

Short-term memory is the gateway to **long-term memory**. We rely on our memory—short- and long-term—to guide everything we do from routine actions to major decisions. Humans have a tremendous capacity for long-term memories, but short-term memory holds only a limited amount and can be overwhelmed by the rapid influx of thoughts during these adolescent years. Is that bad? Not if you can accept the mood fluctuations and confusion you sometimes feel as part of the developing brain's process of growing.

For a practical handle of this complex topic, we usually refer to just short-term memory and long-term memory, which are both processes in forming declarative and non-declarative memories. In short-term memory, we store the information we need at the moment—the rest of a sentence when you are reading, a telephone number, or the name of someone you have just met. This is your "working memory." Information can be held and used in short-term memory for a few seconds or minutes, perhaps hours, until the memory fades or is shifted into the long-term memory. If a short-term memory, such as a phone number, is used frequently, it will be reinforced and can become a long-term memory.

In the process of creating long-term memory, the mind first grasps onto the gist of the information, not every detail. The second step of storing new information is consolidating and organizing it with what has already been stored. This second phase could take several years, during which time the memory may grow weak, new data may change the memory, or the memory may strengthen. Once a memory has been consolidated into long-term memory, it may last a lifetime. For example, a person 50 years old may still remember his first grade teacher's name and what she looked like (a declarative memory). Or a person who has not been on a bicycle in 20 years may be able to hop on a bike and start riding (a nondeclarative memory).

Another example is you score the winning goal in a soccer

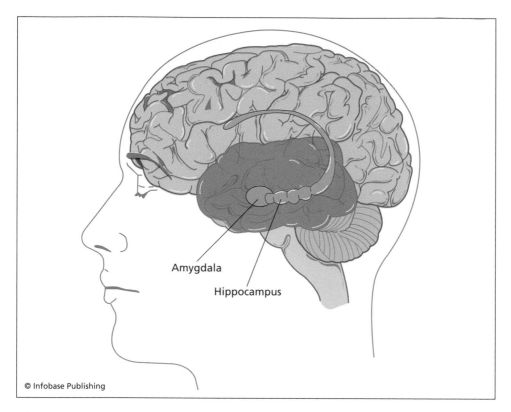

Figure 7.2 **The hippocampus is a critical part of the brain for the storage of memories. The amygdala plays a large role in processing emotions.**

game, the crowds cheer, there is excitement is in the air, and you are the "hero" of the game. You will remember that event for a long time—that is a long-term memory enhanced by emotional memory. But last week, you read a history assignment and got a perfect score on the quiz on specific dates and events, and today you cannot remember those answers. The memory did not "stick." What is the difference? Your brain retains some memories only briefly, others perhaps for a lifetime. Events that evoke strong emotional reactions, either good or bad, are remembered longer. The amygdala is responsible for input in emotional situations (Figure 7.2).

Neuroscientists are beginning to determine the brain circuits and processes responsible for memories. Both long-term and short-term memories come from connections between neurons at the synapses. Back in the 1960s, scientists became aware that genes within the neuron's nucleus played a role in the production of proteins involved in the conversion of short to long-term memory. But how?

You recall that nerve cells communicate by sending impulses through the axon to its end. The impulse triggers the release of chemicals (neurotransmitters) that are transported across the synapse to the target or postsynaptic neuron. The decisive action appears to be at the synapse. Memories are created when nerve cells in a circuit increase the strength of their connections at the synapses. The neurotransmitters that were released by the presynaptic neuron bind to the receptors on the dendrite of the postsynaptic neuron triggering a change in the voltage. This is described as a "firing" of the synapse.

When a synapse fires in brief, high-frequency bursts, a temporary strengthening of the synapse occurs and this is the basis of short-term memory formation. For long-term memories, the synapses must become permanently strengthened. The repeated stimulation, a crucial action at the synapse, seems to activate a protein called **CREB** inside the cell nucleus. CREB turns on genes within the nucleus, setting in motion a series of chemical reactions, which in turn results in the production of "synapse-strengthening" proteins that diffuse throughout the nerve cell. This permanent strengthening of the synapses leads to long-term memories.

THE FRONTAL LOBES

As a person enters adolescence, the biological changes of puberty can overshadow all else at that stage. The adolescent can feel moody—up one minute and down the next, sometimes confused and forgetful. Teens need far more sleep than they usually get and that sometimes affects their alertness and willingness to get up in the mornings. All of these can be critical issues for teenagers and for their parents, too.

In contrast, the biological changes in the brain are primarily unseen on the surface, but are paving the way for new ways of thinking and behaving. While the pruning of unused nerve pathways is progressing, the frontal lobes are undergoing a major increase in myelination of the active nerve fibers going into and out of this executive center of the brain. Beginning in the midteens, the maturing of a ridge in the middle of the frontal lobes controls the ability to maintain attention, focus thoughts more sharply, and handle more complex ways of thinking, such as considering consequences and making choices.

As you enter (or are already into) your teen years, you may want to think about this pruning and the development of your thinking abilities. Remember, you have a lot to say about the way your brain develops. Whatever you are doing—sports or academics or music—those are the abilities that are going to be "hard-wired" as the brain circuits mature.

CONNECTIONS

We have seen how the brain grows and develops from the prenatal stage through adolescence. Some of its growth is genetically predetermined and some of its growth is determined by experiences and the environment. We have considered memory formation, the differences in short-term and long-term memory, and the impact of the protein CREB on the strengthening of long-term memory. In recalling both the growth of neurons and the pruning process, the "use it or lose it" principle reminds us that the choices we make now can affect us throughout our lives.

8

Frontiers
of the Future

Often, advances in medical knowledge are the result of the
study of diseases, and diseases of the brain are some of the most
serious ones. Some problems result from errors in brain development in the prenatal phase, while others begin after birth due to
the effects of malnutrition, trauma and abuse, or accidents. Later,
health habits such as sleep patterns, diet, and exercise can affect
the brain's health. Chronic stress and substance abuse (alcohol,
nicotine, prescription as well as illegal drugs) also affect the health
of the brain.

These problems—both those that we can control, and those
over which we have no control—can have a serious impact. Like
it or not, the growth and development of the brain and nervous
system are involved in every aspect of our lives. The more we

understand how the brain grows and develops, the better we can care for it.

Responding to these challenges, scientists make discoveries, which often open doors to potential brain therapies. The research includes many disciplines, not only biology, chemistry, and physics, but also mathematics and computer science, psychology, and even philosophy and sociology. **Neuroscience** encompasses many areas working together to find ways to cure or repair brain problems and to prevent many of them.

THE CUTTING EDGE OF RESEARCH

Some diseases you cannot cure, but you can make life better for people who have them. Neuroscientists are testing electrical implants to help alleviate injury and disease. One example is cochlear implants for the profoundly deaf, those who cannot be helped by hearing aids (Figure 8.1). Research began more than 40 years ago, but it took a long time and persistent research before cochlear implants were able to provide partial hearing by electrical stimulation of the auditory nerve. A world of sounds—speech and music—is now open to those who before could not hear.

Artificial vision devices are close to becoming available for people who have lost their sight due to diseases of the retina. These devices will enable at least limited vision for many people who are now blind. Work on these devices has been going on since the mid-1980s.

Paralysis occurs in younger as well as older people. The bionic approach, still in development, is a thought-controlled prosthetic device, also known as a brain-machine interface, to use signals from the neurons to stimulate movement. Other

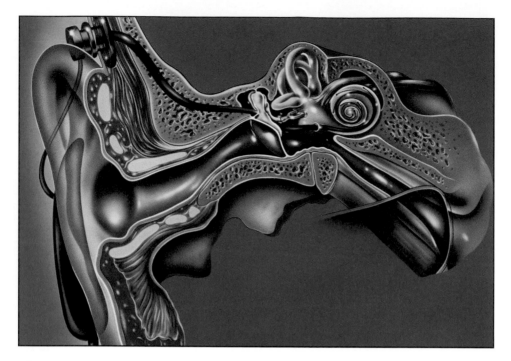

Figure 8.1 A cochlear implant can help restore hearing in the severely deaf.

approaches involve finding a way to stimulate nerve regeneration; that is, new growth of the axons of damaged nerves. The potential of **stem cell** research holds hope for discoveries in this area.

For Parkinson's symptoms, brain pacemakers or deep brain stimulation (DBS) have been approved by U.S. Food and Drug Administration (FDA). Similar to heart pacemakers, a small impulse generator implanted in the chest is connected to electrodes implanted in specific areas of the brain identified with Parkinson's tremors. This technique is being investigated for other neurological disorders, such as epilepsy, as well.

Memory loss is a growing concern, especially the loss caused by Alzheimer's disease. At this point, there are no cures. However, silicon chip implants being tested in rat brains may restore or supplement some functioning of the hippocampus for memory formation and recall. Chemical imbalances of neurotransmitters, especially acetylcholine, seem to be involved in Alzheimer's as well. We have no therapies yet, but research in this direction may prove fruitful in the future.

CONNECTIONS

Research into brain diseases is occurring on many levels. The National Institute of Mental Health (NIMH) and the National Institutes of Health (NIH) are actively investigating a number of areas. One area is the physical basis of memory and learning. Neuroimaging techniques are useful in investigating the role of stress in nerve cell regeneration. Researchers are using these techniques to ask why stress decreases the capacity for growth of new nerve cells, among other questions. Research into the effect of the emotions on thinking processes may lead to the development of new treatments for memory-related disorders. Other research has found that the generation of new nerve cells occurs in the hippocampus, the portion of the brain essential for the formation of memories.

As research continues, some answers, even therapeutic applications will be found, and certainly more questions will arise to challenge us. Throughout it all we know . . .

The brain grows—
by leaps and bounds . . .
with ups and downs . . .

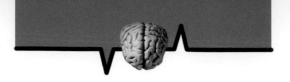

Glossary

Action Potential Also known as the nerve impulse, this occurs when a neuron is activated and temporarily reverses the electrical state of its interior membrane from negative to positive. This nerve impulse travels along the axon to the neuron's terminal, where it triggers the release of neurotransmitters.

Addictive Something that produces an intense, uncontrollable craving that is psychologically or physically habit-forming.

Amygdala Almond-shaped mass located in each of the two temporal lobes. Attaches emotional significance to signals it receives and relays, coordinates information from the senses, alerts fear messages, and interacts with some of the automatic functions of the nervous system such as breathing and heart beat.

Arachnoid Resembling a spider's web.

Astrocytes A type of glial cell that surrounds the brain's capillaries and helps maintain the blood–brain barrier. Astrocytes are also involved in the synaptic process, thought to assist in the reuptake of neurotransmitter molecules after they are released.

Autonomic nervous system The system that controls involuntary actions such as heart rate, breathing, digestion, and glandular functions.

Axon The fiber-like extension from the cell body of a neuron that transmits impulses away from the cell body.

Brain stem A brain structure that connects the brain to the spinal cord. It is made up of the midbrain, the pons, and the medulla. It controls essential "automatic" body functions such as heartbeat, blood pressure, and breathing.

Broca's area Region in the left frontal lobe associated with the movements of mouth, tongue, and larynx that are important for the production of speech.

Cell membrane The thin semipermeable tissue covering that encloses specific portions of a cell.

Cerebellum Located at the back of the brain, it coordinates voluntary skeletal muscle movement, posture, and balance. It may be involved in aspects of motor learning.

Cerebral cortex Thin layer of nerve cells that cover the cerebral hemispheres; responsible for all conscious experience, thought, and planning.

Cerebrospinal fluid (CSF) A liquid within the ventricles of the brain and spinal cord. It provides nourishment to the nerve cells in these areas and circulates to keep pressure equalized.

Cerebrum The large front part of the brain where conscious thought and decision-making occur. It is divided into two cerebral hemispheres, which are in turn divided into four lobes.

Chordates Belong to the phylum Chordata, comprising true vertebrates and those animals having a notochord.

Corpus callosum Thick bundle of nerve fibers (white matter) that connects the left and right cerebral hemispheres.

Cranium The part of the skull that encloses the brain.

CREB A protein designated as a transcription factor inside the cell nucleus. It is responsible for activating synapse-strengthening proteins that transform a short-term memory into a long-term one.

Cytoplasm The contents of a cell, not including the nucleus, cell membrane, axons, and dendrites.

Decibel (dB) Unit for expressing the loudness of sound.

Declarative memory Conscious recall of facts, people, places, and events.

Dendrite Fiber-like extension of a neuron that transmits impulses toward the neuron's cell body.

Dura mater (dura) The tough outer layer of those membranes, the meninges, that cover the brain and spinal cord.

Emotional memory Memory generated by a state of consciousness in which strong feelings, such as joy, sorrow, fear, or hate, color one's experience. These memories often involve the amygdala's alerting the organism to possible "fight or flight" interpretation.

Forebrain The front portion of the three primary divisions of the primitive brain and of the early brain of a vertebrate embryo. It is the largest division of the more developed brain and is credited with the highest intellectual functions.

GABA An amino acid (gamma-aminobutyric acid) that is one of the most widespread neurotransmitters in the brain. Its primary function is to inhibit the firing of neurons.

Ganglion Ganglia (plural) are masses of gray matter existing in the peripheral nervous system.

Glial cells (glia) Support cells for the neurons providing insulation, structural support, and maintaining the environment for the optimum operation of the neuron.

Glutamate The neurotransmitter most widely found in the brain. It excites neurons.

Gyri The ridges or elevated regions in the folds of the convoluted surface of the cerebral cortex. The folds of ridges and fissures provide the cerebral cortex with increased surface area. (Singular form, *gyrus*.)

Hemispheres, right and left The two halves of the cerebrum.

Hindbrain The most posterior portion of the three primary divisions of the brain in the vertebrate embryo.

Hippocampus Essential in memory functions—short-term, and especially long-term. This part of the brain receives and organizes new information.

Hypothalamus Located at the base of forebrain, just under the thalamus, it houses an internal biological clock that generates and regulates the rhythm of cellular activity. It influences hormone secretion, sleep, temperature, thirst, and hunger.

Imaging technology The use of computerized and specialized techniques and instruments to obtain pictures of the interior of the body.

Ion An electrically charged atom or group of atoms formed by the loss or gain of electrons.

Lobe One of the divisions of the brain's cerebral hemisphere.

Long-term memory The part of the brain involved in storing information for longer periods of time, maybe even for a lifetime.

Limbic system A group of inner brain structures involved with emotion, memory, and keeping the body in a steady state (homeostasis).

Membrane The thin covering of a cell or cell part.

Meninges The three membrane coverings of the brain and spinal cord.

Midbrain A small region of the brain stem connecting the cerebrum to the brain stem.

Motor area The region of the brain, stretching in a band across the top from ear-to-ear, that sends impulses to areas of the spinal cord that control muscles and glands.

Myelin The white, fatty substance forming a protective covering (sheath) around axons that insulates them and helps the electrical impulses move more efficiently.

Myelination The process of forming the myelin sheath. It begins around the eighth month in prenatal develop of the human embryo and continues into childhood and later.

Neocortex The site of most of the higher brain functions, it is the largest and evolutionarily most recent portion of the cerebral cortex.

Neural groove A "trench" or fold that forms in the developing fetal brain.

Neural plate A thickening mass that is the first sign of the developing nervous system in the fetal brain.

Neural tube The elongated structure formed when the edges of folded tissue from the neural groove meet. It will become the brain and spinal cord of the embryo.

Neurobiologist A scientist who is concerned with the anatomy and physiology of the nervous system.

Neuromodulator Secondary neurotransmitter that alters the effect of primary neurotransmitters.

Neuroscience The field of study that includes a number of scientific disciplines dealing with the structure, development, function, chemistry, pharmacology, and pathology of the nervous system.

Neuron A nerve cell, the impulse-conducting cell that is the functional unit of the nervous system. In addition to its cell body, neurons have an axon and one or many dendrites.

Neurotransmitter A chemical released by neurons at a synapse for the purpose of transmitting information between neurons via receptors.

Nondeclarative memory Recall without conscious effort. This type of recall is involved in remembering things like skills, habits, and procedural memory.

Notochord A rod-like group of cells that forms the chief axial supporting structure of the body of lower chordates and vertebrate embryos.

Oligodendrocyte A type of glial cell in the central nervous system that wraps itself around an axon forming the myelin sheath. Because of the fatty substance in the oligodendrocytes' membranes, the myelin looks white.

Peripheral nerves Nerves outside of the central nervous system.

Photon A unit of light energy.

Photoreceptors Light sensitive cells in the retina of the eye.

Pia mater (pia) The innermost layer of the meninges, the membranes that cover the brain and spinal cord.

Plasticity Capable of being molded or reshaped.

Postsynaptic neuron The neuron receiving information via a neurotransmitter across a synapse.

Presynaptic neuron The neuron sending information via a neurotransmitter across a synapse.

Purkinje cells Neurons of the cerebellum.

Prune To cut away unused nerve pathways to achieve a more stable system.

Refinement phase The period of time when the system is undergoing finer, more exacting distinctions, as in fine-tuning.

Reflex loop A nerve pathway from sensory neuron to interneuron to motor neuron involved in a quick response to a stimulus.

Reflex A rapid, automatic response to a stimulus that does not involve a message to the brain; it is controlled by the spinal cord.

Resting potential The difference in electrical charge between the inside and outside of an undisturbed, unstimulated nerve cell membrane.

Reticular formation A complex of nerve cells located in the brain stem that filters the incoming messages, preventing an overload of stimuli from passing on through the system.

Selective permeability The process by which only certain substances are allowed to pass through a membrane.

Sensory cortex That area of the cerebral cortex that receives and interprets sensory nerve impulses.

Sensory memory Information from the eyes, ears, and other senses that is held by the brain for a short time until it is incorporated into other types memory or discarded.

Short-term memory The "working memory" where the brain temporarily stores information needed at the moment.

Spinal cord Nerve tissue that extends downward from the brain stem through the vertebral column (backbone).

Stem cells Undifferentiated (not specialized) cells that have the ability to undergo cell division and become specialized cells, such as a neuron, skin cell, or heart cell.

Sulci The fissures in the folds of the convoluted surface of the cerebral cortex that allow the cerebral cortex's surface area to fold in upon itself, thus increasing surface area. (Singular form, *sulcus*.)

Sutures The juncture or line of closing between two parts.

Synapse The area between the end of the axon and the dendrite of the adjacent cell over which neurotransmitters must be transmitted.

Thalamus A major clearinghouse or gateway for information going to and from the spinal cord and the cerebrum. It receives all sensory impulses except those associated with the sense of smell. It channels these signals to the appropriate region of the cerebral cortex for interpretation.

Threshold The minimum level of stimulation necessary to activate a neuron.

Ventricles Fluid-filled spaces in the brain.

Vesicles Small pouches at the ends of the axons in which neurotransmitters are stored.

Wernicke's area A brain region responsible for the comprehension of language and the production of meaningful speech.

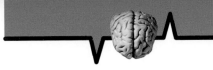

Bibliography

BOOKS

Atwater, Mary. *The Animal Kingdom*. New York: Macmillan/ McGraw-Hill School Publishing, 1993.

Barmeier, Jim. *The Brain*. San Diego, Calif.: Lucent Books, 1996.

Barrett, Susan. *It's All in Your Head: A Guide to Understanding Your Brain and Boosting Your Brain Power*. Minneapolis, Minn.: Free Spirit Publishing, 1992.

Bergen, Doris, and Juliet Coscia. *Brain Research and Childhood Education—Implications for Educators*. Olney, Md.: Association for Childhood Education International, 2001.

Bloom, Floyd E., M. Flint Beal, and David J. Kupfer (editors). *The Dana Guide to Brain Health*. New York: The Free Press, Simon & Schuster, 2003.

Brynie, Faith Hickman. *The Physical Brain*. Woodbridge, Conn.: Blackbirch Press, 2001.

Brynie, Faith Hickman. *101 Questions Your Brain Has Asked About Itself But Couldn't Answer Until Now*. Brookfield, Conn.: The Millbrook Press, 1998.

Carey, Joseph (editor). *Brain Facts: A Primer on the Brain and Nervous System*. Washington, D.C.: Society for Neuroscience, 2002.

Carter, Rita. *Mapping the Mind*. Berkeley, Calif.: University of California Press, 1998.

Eliot, Lise, Ph.D. *What's Going On in There?* New York: Bantam Books, 1999.

Fortin, Francois. *Major Systems of the Body*. Milwaukee, Wis.: World Almanac Library, 2002.

Greenfield, Susan. *The Human Brain: A Guided Tour*. New York: Basic Books, 1997.

Greenfield, Susan. *The Private Life of the Brain: Emotions, Consciousness, and the Secret of the Self*. New York: John Wiley & Sons, 2000.

Hayhurst, Chris. *The Brain and Spinal Cord—Learning How We Think, Feel, and Move*. New York: Rosen Publishing Group, 2002.

Kandel, Eric R., James H. Schwartz, Thomas M. Jessell (eds). *Principles of Neural Science*, 4th ed. New York: McGraw-Hill, Health Professions Division, 2000.

Kapp, Loren. *Perspectives in Human Biology*. Belmont, Calif.: Wadsworth Publishing, 1998.

Kotulak, Ronald. *Inside the Brain: Revolutionary Discoveries of How the Mind Works*. Kansas City, Mo.: Andrews and McMeel, 1996.

Kuffler, Stephen W., John G. Nicholls, and A. Robert Martin. *From Neuron to Brain*, 2nd ed. Sunderland, Mass.: Sinauer Associates, 1984.

Lambert, Mark. *The Brain and Nervous System*. Englewood Cliffs, N.J.: Silver Burdett Press, 1988.

LeDoux, Joseph. *Synaptic Self: How Our Brains Become Who We Are*. New York: Viking Penguin Putnam, 2002.

Light, Douglas. *The Senses*. Philadelphia: Chelsea House Publishers, 2005.

Mathers, Douglas. *Brain: You and Your Body Series*. Mahwah, N.J.: Troll Associates Publishers, 1992.

McGaugh, James A. *Memory and Emotion*. New York: Columbia University Press, 2003.

Miller, Kenneth, and Joseph Levine. *Biology*. Upper Saddle River, N.J.: Pearson/Prentice Hall, 2004.

Moffett, Shannon. *The Three-Pound Enigma: The Human Brain and the Quest to Unlock Its Mysteries*. Chapel Hill, N.C.: Algonquin Books, 2006.

National Geographic Education Division, and Alton Biggs, et al. *Life Sciences*. Columbus, Ohio: Glencoe/McGraw-Hill, 2005.

Netter, Frank H., M.D. *Nervous System: The CIBA Collection of Medical Illustrations, Vol. 1*. New York: CIBA Pharmaceutical Products, 1958.

Newquest, H.P. *The Great Brain Book: An Inside Look at the Inside of Your Head*. New York: Scholastic, Inc., 2004.

Papalia, Diane E., and Sally Wendkos Olds. *Human Development*. New York: McGraw-Hill, 1995.

Parker, Steve. *The Brain and Nervous System*. Danbury, Conn.: Franklin Watts, 1990.

Powledge, Tabitha M. *Your Brain: How You Got It and How It Works*. New York: Charles Scribner's Sons, 1994.

Restak, Richard M. *The Secret Life of the Brain*. The Dana Press/ Joseph Henry Press, 2001.

Rowan, Pete. *Big Head*. New York: Alfred A. Knopf, 1998.

Shier, David, Jackie Butler, and Ricki Lewis. *Hole's Human Anatomy and Physiology*, 7th ed. Dubuque, Iowa: William C. Brown Publishers, 1996.

Siegel, Daniel. *The Developing Mind: Toward a Neurobiology of Interpersonal Experience*. New York: Guilford Press, 1999.

Simon, Seymour. *The Brain: Our Nervous System*. New York: Morrow Junior Books, 1997.

Silverstein, Alvin, and Virginia Silverstein. *World of the Brain*. New York: William Morrow, 1986.

Silverstein, Alvin, Virginia Silverstein, and Robert Silverstein. *The Nervous System*. New York: Twenty-First Century Books, Henry Holt, 1994.

Squire, Larry R., and Eric R. Kandel. *Memory: From Mind to Molecules*. New York: Scientific American Library, 1999.

Strauch, Barbara. *The Primal Teen: What the New Discoveries About the Teenage Brain Tell Us About our Kids*. New York: Doubleday, 2003.

Trefil, James. *Are We Unique?* New York: John Wiley & Sons, 1997.

Yepsen, Roger. *Smarten Up! How to Increase Your Brain Power*. Boston: Little, Brown, 1990.

ARTICLES

Anderson, B., and T. Harvey. "Alterations in Cortical Thickness and Neuronal Density in the Frontal Cortex of Albert Einstein." *Neuroscience Letters* 210 (1996): 161–164.

Ariniello, Leah. *Brain Briefings*. Society for Neuroscience, Washington, D.C. Available online. URL: http://www.sfn.org/index.cfm?pagename=brainBriefings_chrolongical.

Ariniello, Leah. *Brain Backgrounders*. Society for Neuroscience, Washington, D.C. Available online. URL: http://www.sfn.org/index.cfm?pagename=brainBackgrounders_main.

Best, Ben. "Brain Neurotransmitters." Available online. URL: http://www.benbest.com/science/anatmind/anatmd10.html.

Bishop, Bill. "Your Brain on Drugs." *DANA Foundation Newsletter* 12:10 (2005): 7.

Cahill, Larry. "His Brain, Her Brain: Sex-Linked Brain Differences." *Scientific American* (May 2005). Available online. URL: http://healthfully.org/medicalscience/id8.html.

Chudler, Eric, Ph.D. "A Computer in Your Head." *Odyssey* 10 (March 2001): 6–7.

Chudler, Eric, Ph.D. "She Brains—He Brains." *Neuroscience Education*. Available online. URL: http://faculty.washington.edu/chudler/heshe.html.

Chudler, Eric, Ph.D. "Discovery of Neurotransmitters." *Neuroscience Education*. Available online. URL: http://faculty.washington.edu/chudler/chnt1.html.

Chudler, Eric, Ph.D. "Brain Development." *Neuroscience Education*. Available online. URL: http://faculty.washington.edu/chudler/dev.html.

Darnell, Robert B. "Controlling the Synapse—49 Proteins at a Time." *Howard Hughes Medical Institute (HHMI) Newsletter* (July 24, 2005). Available online. URL: http://hhmi.org/news/darnell2.html.

DeFrancesco, Laura. "Watching How the Brain Grows—MRI Offers New Insight Into Brain Development." *The Scientist* 16:3 (2002): 27.

Diamond, M.C., A.B. Scheibel, G.M. Murphy, Jr., and T. Harvey. "On the Brain of a Scientist: Albert Einstein." *Experimental Neurology* 88 (1985): 198–204.

Fields, R. Douglas. "Making Memories Stick." *Scientific American* (February 2005): 75–81.

Freudenrich, Craig C. "How Your Brain Works." *How Stuff Works*. Available online. URL: http://science.howstuffworks.com/brain. htm.

Giedd, Jay N., et al. "Brain Development During Childhood and Adolescence: A Longitudinal MRI Study." *Nature Neuroscience* 2:10 (1999): 861–863.

Horgan, John. "Brain." *Discover* (October 2005): 36–37.

Howard Florey Institute of Experimental Physiology and Medicine. "Getting Our Heads Around the Brain—Neurotransmitters and Drugs." PBS *NOVA Science in the News*. Available online. URL: http://www.science.org.au/nova/040/040box04.htm.

Kuwana, Ellen. "Women Have More Frontal Lobe Neurons Than Men." *Neuroscience for Kids*. Available online. URL: http://faculty.washington.edu/chudler/wome.html.

LaRossa, Maureen Mulligan, R.N., and Sheena L. Carter, Ph.D. "Understanding How the Brain Develops." Emory University School of Medicine, Department of Pediatrics. Available online. URL: http://med.emory.edu/neonatology/dpc/brain.htm. Revised February 7, 2005.

Lorain, Peter. "Brain Development in Young Adolescents." Available online. URL: http://www.nea.org/teachexperience/msk030110. html.

MacDonald, Ann. "Deep Brain Stimulation: A Technique for Mood, Too?" *Brain Work—The Neuroscience Newsletter* 15:5 (2005): 1–4.

"Mapping the Mysteries of the Mind." Available online. URL: http://www.mcmaster.ca/ua/opr/times/fall98/witelson.htm.

Massimini, Marcello, et al. "Breakdown of Cortical Effective Connectivity During Sleep." *Science* 309 (2005): 2228–2232.

McManus, Rich. "Summer Lecture Series Provokes Young Minds." Reported in *The NIH Record* LV:15 (July 22, 2003). Available online. URL: http://www.nih.gov/news/NIH-Record/07_22_2003/story03.htm.

Miller, Greg. "Mutant Mice Reveal Secrets of the Brain's Impressionable Youth." *Science* 309 (2005): 2145.

National Institute of Mental Health. "Cognitive Research at the National Institute of Mental Health." Archived publication, 2000. Available online. URL: http://mentalhealth.about.com/library/rs/blcog.htm.

National Institute of Mental Health. *Teenage Brain: A Work in Progress.* National Institute of Mental Health, NIH Publication No. 01-4929. Bethesda, Md.: National Institutes of Health, 2004. Available online. URL: www.mentalhealth.gov/publicat/teenbrain.cfm.

National Institute of Mental Health. "Imaging Study Shows Brain Maturing." National Institute of Mental Health press release (May 17, 2004). Available online. URL: http://www.eurekalert.org/pub_releases/2004-05/niom-iss051304.php.

National Institute of Neurological Disorders and Stroke (NINDS). "Brain Basics: Know Your Brain." NINDS Brain Resources and Information Network (BRAIN) (February 9, 2005). Available online. URL: http://www.ninds.nih.gov/disorders/brain_basics/know_your_brain.htm.

Olsen, Steve. "Memory Circuits." *Howard Hughes Medical Institute (HHMI) Bulletin* (Fall 2004): 14–23. Available online. URL: http://hhmi.org/bulletin/fall2004/synapses/.

Pascual, Olivier, Kristen B. Casper, Cathryn Kubera, et al. "Astrocytic Purinergic Signaling Coordinates Synaptic Networks." *Science* 310 (2005): 113–116.

Patoine, Brenda. "Rethinking the Synapse: Emerging Science Challenges Old Assumptions." *Brain Work—The Neuroscience Newsletter* 15:6 (2005): 1–5.

PBS *Frontline*. "Inside the Teenage Brain." Available online. URL: http://www.pbs.org/wgbh/pages/frontline/shows/teenbrain/.

"Profile: Dr. Sandra Witelson." Available online. URL: http://www.science.ca/scientists/scientistprofile.php?pID=273.

Recer, Paul. "Researchers Find Difference in Gays." Associated Press (March 2, 1998). *We Are Family*. Available online. URL: http://www.waf.org/familyarchives/orientation/studies/Researchers%20Find%20Difference%20in%20Gays.htm.

Scheibel, Arnold B., M.D. *Embryological Development of the Human Brain*. Seattle, Wash.: New Horizons for Learning, 2002.

Suplee, Curt. "Key Brain Growth Goes on Into Teens—Study Disputes Old Assumptions." *Washington Post* (March 8, 2000). Available online. URL: http://www.washingtonpost.com/ac2/wp-dyn?pagename=article&node=&contentId=A35524-2000Mar8.

Thiebaut de Schotten, Michel, Marika Urbanski, Hugues Duffau, et al. "Direct Evidence of a Parietal-Frontal Pathway Subserving Spatial Awareness in Humans." *Science* 309 (2005): 2226–2228.

Thompson, Paul M., et al. "Growth Patterns in the Developing Brain Detected by Using Continuum Mechanical Tensor Maps." *Nature* 404 (2000): 190–193.

Toland, Bill. "Doctor Kept Einstein's Brain in Jar 43 Years." *Pittsburg Post-Gazette* (April 17, 2005). Available online. URL: http://www.post-gazette.com/pg/05107/488975.stm.

Volkow, Nora D. "Drug Addiction: Why the Brain Loses Control." Lecture Series on the Brain, Learning and Memory, University of California–Irvine, January 2002.

Witelson, S.F., D.L. Kigar, and T. Harvey. "The Exceptional Brain of Albert Einstein." *The Lancet* 353 (1999): 2149–2153.

Zelazo, Philip David, Ph.D. "Brain Growth and the Development of Executive Function." *About Kids' Health*. Available online. URL: http://www.aboutkidshealth.ca.

Zelazo, Philip David, Ph.D. "What is Executive Function?" *About Kids' Health*. Available online. URL: http://www.aboutkidshealth.ca.

Further Reading

Bloom, Floyd E., M. Flint Beal, and David J. Kupfer (editors). *The Dana Guide to Brain Health*. New York: The Free Press, Simon & Schuster, 2003.

Brynie, Faith Hickman. *The Physical Brain*. Woodbridge, Conn.: Blackbirch Press, 2001.

Carey, Joseph (editor). *Brain Facts: A Primer on the Brain and Nervous System*. Washington, D.C.: Society for Neuroscience, 2002.

McGaugh, James A. *Memory and Emotion*. New York: Columbia University Press, 2003.

Newquest, H.P. *The Great Brain Book: An Inside Look at the Inside of Your Head*. New York: Scholastic, Inc., 2004.

Restak, Richard M. *The Secret Life of the Brain*. The Dana Press/ Joseph Henry Press, 2001.

Strauch, Barbara. *The Primal Teen: What the New Discoveries About the Teenage Brain Tell Us About our Kids*. New York: Doubleday, 2003.

WEB SITES

Neuroscience for Kids
http://faculty.washington.edu/chudler/neurok.html
Professor Eric Chudler of the University of Washington has gathered this extensive list of neuroscience Web sites. With over 150 links, and more being added all the time, you are sure to find information on any topic related to the brain at this site.

Dana BrainWeb

http://www.dana.org/brainweb/

The Dana Alliance for the Brain is a nonprofit organization of over 200 pre-eminent brain scientists. Dana's Web site provides a huge amount of information on the human brain, including book lists, glossaries, overviews of current research, and articles on new developments in the field of neuroscience.

National Institute of Mental Health (NIMH) and National Institutes of Health (NIH)

http://www.nimh.nih.gov/publicat/pubListing.cfm?dID=44

Neuroscience publication topics may be found at this site as well as links to other health topics. Scan the different topics as well as the available topics under each.

Inside the Teenage Brain

http://www.pbs.org/wgbh/pages/frontline/shows/teenbrain/

This excellent site is a companion to an episode that appeared on the television program *Frontline*.

Society for Neuroscience

http://web.sfn.org

Click on "Publications." Then choose "Brain Briefings," "Brain Backgrounders," or "Brain Facts."

Washington University School of Medicine. Neuroscience Tutorial

http://thalamus.wustl.edu/course/

The Washington University School of Medicine offers this illustrated tutorial on the anatomy of the human brain. Created in conjunction with the University's first-year course for medical students, the site provides detailed information on all the basics of clinical neuroscience.

Picture Credits

page:

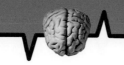

Index

About the Authors

Ann McIntosh Hoffelder, Ph.D., has been fascinated with the potential of the human brain for many years. From her first dissection of lab animals as a ninth grader to her current research in neurology, Dr. Hoffelder's professional life has been in teaching chemistry, primarily at the college/university level. During her tenure as professor and department chair in chemistry at Cumberland College, Dr. Ann (as her students called her) received Outstanding Teacher awards from fellow faculty and students.

Along with an intense interest in the development of the human brain, **Robert L. Hoffelder, Ph.D.**, devotes time to evolutionary and anthropological studies, especially in the interrelating of the physical, biological, and social sciences. Prior to his professional life as professor and department chair in Sociology at Cumberland College, he was a civilian personnel officer at the Navy Electronics Laboratory, San Diego. The Hoffelders live in Laguna Woods, California.

ABOUT THE EDITOR

Eric H. Chudler, Ph.D., is a research neuroscientist who has investigated the brain mechanisms of pain and nociception since 1978. Dr. Chudler received his Ph.D. from the Department of Psychology at the University of Washington in Seattle. He is currently a research associate professor in the University of Washington Department of Bioengineering and director of education and outreach at University of Washington Engineered Biomaterials.